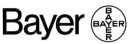

Bayer

Pharmaceutical Division

Richard K. Goodstein, M.D.
Vice President
Scientific Relations

Dear Doctor:

Thank you for taking time out to reply to the recent mail that we sent to your office.

In celebration of the millennium, Bayer Corporation, Pharmaceutical Division, maker of Cipro® (ciprofloxacin HCl) Tablets, Cipro® (ciprofloxacin) 5% and 10% Oral Suspension, and Cipro® I.V. (ciprofloxacin), wishes to present you with this volume on the history of medicine and medical pioneers over the last 1000 years.

The Medical Millennium: 1000 Pioneers Who Have Contributed to the Development of Medicine Over the Last 1000 Years

This encyclopedic volume covers the vast knowledge accumulated through the centuries by physicians and surgeons. The rich illustrations are sure to provide you with hours of delightful reading and informative study.

We are sure that this will be a welcome addition to your library.

Cordially,

Richard K. Goodstein, M.D.
Vice President, Scientific Relations

Bayer Corporation
400 Morgan Lane
West Haven, CT 06516-4175
Phone 203 812-6592
Fax 203 812-6547

The Medical Millennium

The Medical Millennium

1000 pioneers who have contributed to the development of medicine over the last 1000 years

H.S.J. Lee

The Parthenon Publishing Group

International Publishers in Medicine, Science & Technology

NEW YORK   LONDON

Published in the USA by
The Parthenon Publishing Group Inc.
One Blue Hill Plaza
PO Box 1564, Pearl River
New York 10965, USA

Published in the UK by
The Parthenon Publishing Group Limited
Casterton Hall, Carnforth
Lancs. LA6 2LA, UK

British Library Cataloging in Publication Data

The medical millennium
  1. Physicians - Biography - Dictionaries 2. Medicine -
  History
  I . Lee, H. S. J.
  610 . 9 ' 22

  ISBN: 1-85070-466-X

Library of Congress Cataloging-in-Publication Data

The medical millennium / edited by H.S.J. Lee
    p. ; cm
  ISBN 1-85070-466-X (alk. paper)
  1. Medicine--History--Encyclopedias. 2. Surgery--History--Encyclopedias. I. Lee, H.
S. J.
  [DNLM: 1. Physicians--Biography. 2. History of Medicine--Biography. 3.
Science--Biography. 4. Surgery--Biography. WZ 112 M4895 1999]
  R125 M413 1999
  610'.9--dc21
                                                                99-044527

Typesetting by H&H Graphics, Blackburn, UK
Printed and bound by The Bath Press, Bath, UK

Foreword

Although throughout antiquity there was a considerable interest in the concept of medical care, modern medicine (based as it is on a scientific understanding of the human body) is entirely a product of the last millennium. Whilst the vast majority of advances in the field have taken place in relatively recent times, the origins of these advances can often be traced to an earlier period in the millennium.

The objective of this book is to identify and describe some of the men and women who have made an especially notable contribution to medical advances throughout the last 1000 years. Since so many people in so many places over so many years have made important contributions to our knowledge of the human body and our understanding of medicine itself, it is a particularly challenging task to try to identify just 1000 names. Some entries would be universally agreed upon – Louis Pasteur, James Harvey or Jonas Salk are all obvious examples. But the choice of many other key contributors to the science is bound to be, to some extent, personal and arbitrary.

In this book the reader will find descriptions of many of the most important contributions to modern medicine – they marked the path of progress that others follow. Nevertheless, I freely acknowledge that many others deserve to be added to the role of honor and I welcome suggestions for a future – and enlarged – edition. In the meantime, I trust that this volume will provide an interesting and useful resource and an aide-mémoire for all those interested in the practice and history of medicine.

Helen S. J. Lee
January 2000

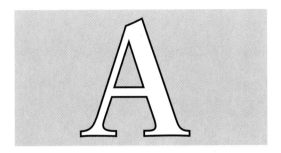

Peter of Abano

(1250–1316) Italian polymath who attempted to reconcile Greek, Arab and Jewish medical practice in his *Conciliator*, he studied and classified poisons and was subjected to the Inquisition.

Haly Abbas

(d 994) Arab physician who described goiter, malignant anthrax, smallpox, gave contraceptive advice, and wrote *Almaleki*.

John Jacob Abel

(1857–1938) American hematologist and biochemist, who was the first to use an artificial membrane in pioneering work on renal dialysis, developed plasmapherisis, extracted epinephrine, and crystallized insulin.

John Abernethy

(1764–1831) British surgeon who was the first to ligate the external iliac artery for aneurysm, and improved treatment of lumbar abscesses by incising with minimal exposure to air.

Sir Edward Penley Abraham

(b 1913) British biochemist who developed crystalline sodium salt of penicillin, thus confirming its purity, and also isolated cephalosporin C.

Alessandro Achillini

(1463–1512) Italian anatomist who discovered the malleus, incus, labyrinth and ileocecal valve.

Joseph Adams

(1756–1818) British physician and early endocrinogist who, in 1814, published *Supposed Hereditary Properties of Disease*, described gout, scrofula and goiter in cretinism.

Robert Adams

(1791–1875) Irish physician and surgeon who a gave classic accounts of essential heart block and rheumatic gout, and was first to distinguish osteo- from rheumatoid arthritis.

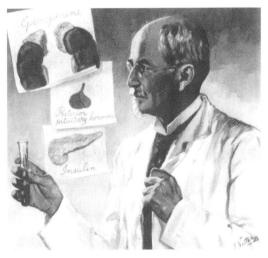

John Jacob Abel

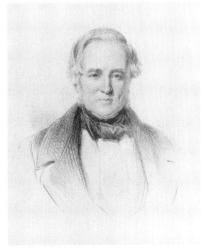

Robert Adams

Thomas Addison

(1793–1860) British endocrinologist and urologist who, in 1855, wrote *On the Constitutional and Local Effects of Disease of the Suprarenal Capsules*, and described pernicious anemia.

Edgar Douglas Adrian

(1889–1977) British neurophysiologist who developed the all-or-none law of nerve impulse transmission, Nobel laureate in 1932, and wrote *The Physical Background of Perception* (1947).

Paul of Aegina

(625–690) Famous Greek physician and surgeon who treated fractures and dislocations, performed tracheotomy, mastectomy for tumor, trephination of the skull and surgical treatment of hernia.

Aesculapius

(c 1250 BC) Ancient Greek physician, mentioned in Homer's *Iliad*, said to be the son of the god Apollo and Coronis, his origin is unknown but his name is synonymous with medicine and temples were built to him throughout Greece.

Raymond Perry Ahlquist

(1914–1983) American pharmacologist who the studied biological actions of epinephrine and norepinephrine and showed them to be due to differential sensitivities of alpha and beta cell receptors.

Albertus Magnus

(1200–1280) German philosopher and cleric and the most eminent naturalist of the thirteenth century, he recommended powdered hog testes for impotence, and powdered hare womb for infertile women, and gave a detailed description of arsenic.

Bernhard Siegfried Albinus

(1697–1770) Important German anatomist and obstetrician and a great anatomic illustrator, produced atlases on bones, muscles, veins, arteries, intestines, the fetal skeleton, and the gravid uterus.

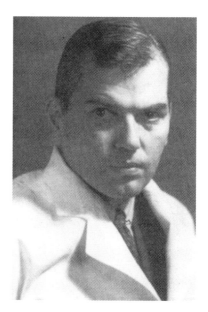

Fuller Albright

Fuller Albright

(1900–1969) American endocrinologist and hematologist who described hyperparathyroidism, and studied calcium metabolism and bone disorders.

Albucasis

(c 936–1013) Spanish physician and surgeon who wrote *At-Tasrif*, which mentions operations for elephantiasis and goiter. He described surgical instruments, lithotomy, paralysis in spinal fracture, wrote on fractures and dislocations, and described congenital deformities and hemophilia.

Ludwig Alder

(1876–1958) Austrian endocrinologist and gynecologist who studied cyclical changes in the endometrium.

Jean Louis Alibert

(1768–1837) French physician and the founder of dermatology who gave the first description of mycosis fungoides, keloid, leishmaniasis, and introduced the terms syphilis and dermatosis.

Edgar Allen

(1892–1943) American endocrinologist and gynecologist who, in 1927, showed that the onset of menstruation occurs when estrogen stops acting on the endometrium.

Sidney Altman

(b 1939) Canadian molecular biologist and Nobel laureate who studied RNA transcription and its cleavage by ribonuclease P.

Roger E C Altounyan

(1922–1987) British physician who invented the anti-asthma drug Intal and the spinhaler device.

Alois Alzheimer

(1864–1915) German neurologist who described presenile dementia, and perfected a stain for the Negri bodies of rabies.

William Anderson

(1842–1900) British urologist remembered for his contribution to recognizing Anderson-Fabry disease (burning sensation in hands and feet, dark nodular skin lesions and renal failure) in 1839.

Gabriel Andral

(1797–1876) French physician who was the first to suggest the importance of chemical examination of blood in morbid conditions, wrote an important work on anemia, and was the founder of clinical hematology.

Nicolas André

(1658–1742) French physician and surgeon who coined the term orthopedics, was first to describe infra-orbital neuralgia, and wrote *Orthopedics, or the art of preventing and correcting bodily deformities in children*, in 1741.

Christian Boehmer Anfinsen

(1916–1995) American biochemist and Nobel laureate who developed methods for enzymic and chemical hydrolysis of proteins and chromatographic identification of peptides, and elucidated the structure of ribonuclease.

Gilbertus Anglicus

(1180–1250) British physician who gave original accounts of leprosy and smallpox, directions on hygiene for travelers, and claimed that sexual excess weakened joints and could lead to arthritis.

Hieronymus Fabricius ab Aquapendente

(1537–1619) Italian surgeon, gynecologist and anatomist who wrote on the female reproductive apparatus, produced the first drawing of the corpus luteum, described spinal curvature, valves in veins, wry neck and club foot, and wrote *De formato foetu and De foratione ovi et pulli*.

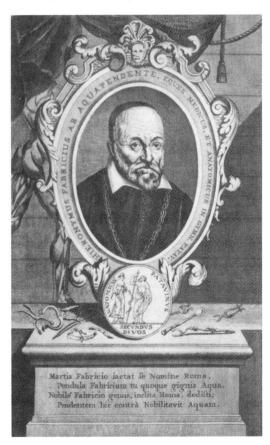

Hieronymus Fabricius ab Aquapendente

Werner Arber

(b 1929) Swiss microbiologist who studied bacteriophages and bacterial defense against them using restriction enzymes to cut the phage DNA at specific points, leading to an opening into the new field of genetic engineering.

Giovanni Arcolani

(d 1484) Early Italian dentist and mouth surgeon who developed aural syringes and flexible catheters, and filled teeth with gold leaf.

John of Arderne

(1306–1380) First great British surgeon who operated on fistula in ano, appendicitis, described gout, tetanus and carcinoma, and devised instruments for clysters (enemas).

Douglas Argyll Robertson

(1837–1909) British ophthalmologist who studied the etiology of glaucoma, retinitis pigmentosa, diphtheritic ophthalmia and buphthalamus, and described the classic sign of neurosyphilis of small, irregular, unequal pupils which constrict on accommodation but not in response to light.

Charles N Armstrong

(b 1897) British endocrinologist and neurologist who successfully treated myxedema with extract of sheep thyroid.

Bernhardt Aschner

(1883–1960) Austrian endocrinologist who discovered the oculocardiac reflex, created long-lived hypophysectomized dogs to study the pituitary, and wrote *Endocrine Disorders of Females and Constitutional Therapy*.

Ludwig Aschoff

(1866–1942) Skilled German pathologist who studied the heart and acute rheumatic fever, and identified a specific valvular lesion which he also found in subcutaneous nodules, joints, tendons, the aorta and pleura. He also developed the concept of the reticuloendothelial system.

Gaspare Aselli

(1581–1626) Italian physician and anatomist who discovered the lacteal (lymphatic) vessels of the intestine, studied the action of poisons, recurring calculi and fistula-in-ano.

Winifred Ashby

(1879–1975) American hematologist who developed techniques for estimating red cell survival rates, diagnostic tests for syphilis, and studied carbonic anhydrase in the brain.

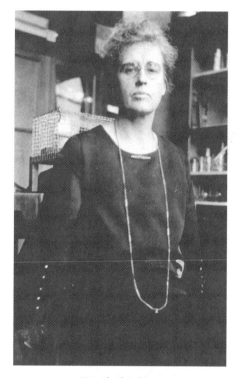

Winifred Ashby

Jean Astruc

(1684–1766) French physician who contributed to many aspects of medicine including venereology, midwifery, and childhood diseases.

Leopold Auenbrugger

(1722–1809) Austrian physician who first used and described percussion of the chest in diagnosis.

Charlotte Auerbach

(1899–1994) German-born British biochemist who discovered chemical mutagenesis and compared the differences between the actions of chemical mutagens and X-rays.

Gerald D Auerbach

(1927–1991) American endocrinologist who was the first to isolate parathyroid hormone.

Avenzoar

(c 1072–1162) Spanish physician who wrote *Rectification of Health*, was the first to test medicines on animals, described tracheotomy, mediastinal tumor, kidney stones, and pericarditis.

Oswald Theodore Avery

(1877–1955) American microbiologist who studied rough and smooth strains of pneumococci and the transformation from the former to the virulent smooth strain by the presence of DNA from dead bacteria.

Avicenna

(980–1037) Arab physician, called the prince of physicians, who wrote an enormous and influential *Canon of Medicine*. He described diabetes mellitus, contraception, anthrax, epilepsy, dementia, headache, pleurisy, advised freshening of ununited fractures, and recognized the contagiousness of tuberculosis.

Richard Axel

(b 1946) American molecular biologist who showed that DNA can be cleaved by staphylococcal nucleases in certain regions of active genes, and used this technique in tissue culture to add viral genes to produce mutations and determine the effect on gene activity.

Julius Axelrod

(b 1912) American neurologist and biochemist, Nobel laureate in 1970, who studied the action of neurotransmitters, schizophrenia, and circadian rhythms.

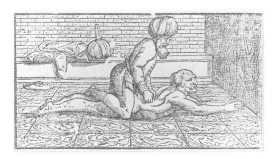

Avicenna applying massage

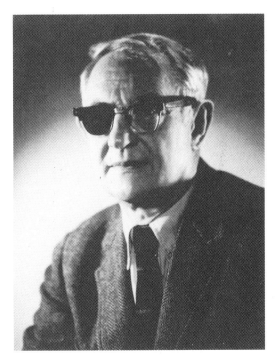

Julius Axelrod

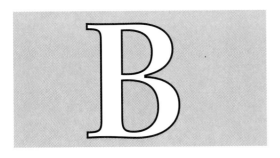

Joseph FF Babinski

(1857–1932) French neurologist who described the extensor plantar reflex characteristic of an upper motor neurone lesion, adiposogenital dystrophy, and lesions of the pontobulbar region.

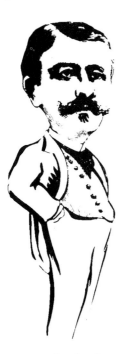

Joseph Babinski

Roger Bacon

(1214–1294) Great British experimenter of his century, mathematician, astronomer, chemist and physician, who reformed the calendar, studied lenses and vision.

Karl Ernst von Baer

(1792–1876) Estonian embryologist who, in 1827, published his discovery of the mammalian ovum. He also described the germ layers, the notochord and the neural tube in the embryo.

William S Baer

(1872–1931) American orthopedic surgeon who used a membrane from pig bladder in arthroplasty. He also treated chronic osteomyelitis with maggots (before antibiotics).

Giorgio Baglivi

(1668–1706) Italian anatomist who was the first to distinguish between smooth and striped muscle.

Matthew Baillie

(1761–1823) British physician who wrote *Morbid Anatomy* (1793), correlated case history with autopsy, and was the first to attempt to treat pathology as a separate subject.

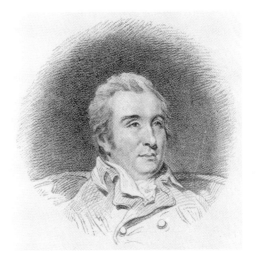

Matthew Baillie

Guillaume de Baillou

(1538–1616) French physician and the first epidemiologist of modern times, he gave the first description of whooping cough, diphtheria and acute rheumatic fever, introduced the word rheumatism and wrote the first treatise on arthritis. He also studied measles, typhus, plague and smallpox.

Samuel Baird

(1742–1821) American physician who wrote an essay on diphtheria or 'angina suffocativa' in 1771.

Sir George Baker

(1722–1809) British physician who first described Devonshire colic (lead poisoning).

Sir Charles A Ballance

(1856–1936) British surgeon who pioneered nerve grafting, the management of intracranial complications of middle ear disease, and mastoid surgery.

David Baltimore

(b 1938) American molecular biologist and Nobel laureate who worked on viral genetics, and discovered reverse transcriptase, now used to manipulate the genetic code.

Sir Roger G Bannister

(b 1929) British neurologist and athlete who studied the physiology of exercise, and edited *Brain's Clinical Neurology* from 1969.

Guido Banti

(1852–1925) Notable Italian pathologist and bacteriologist who described Banti syndrome of splenomegaly with nonleukemic anemia.

Sir Frederick G Banting

(1891–1941) Canadian endocrinologist and Nobel laureate in 1923 for his discovery of insulin.

Robert Bárány

(1876–1936) Austrian otologist and Nobel laureate who studied the balancing apparatus of the inner ear and its connection to the brain.

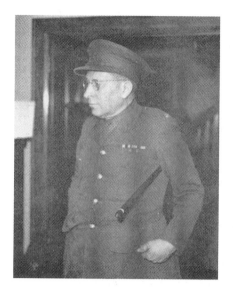

Frederick Banting

Sir Joseph Barcroft

(1872–1947) Irish-born British physiologist who studied respiratory function, especially under extreme conditions, binding and dissociation of O_2 in hemoglobin, and fetal metabolism.

Samuel Bard

(1742–1821) American physician and obstetrician who was instrumental in the founding of the New York Hospital and wrote treatises on midwifery and on diphtheria.

Christiaan Neethling Barnard

(b 1922) South African heart surgeon who performed the first successful human heart transplant.

Caspar Bartholin, elder

(1585–1629) Danish physician who described a 'humor' in the cavity of the adrenals which was passed to the kidneys and then the urine. He was the first to describe the functions of the olfactory nerve and was the author of *Anatomicae Institutiones Corporis Humani* (1611).

Caspar Bartholin, younger

(1655–1738) Danish anatomist who gave the first description of the greater vestibular glands in the female reproductive system, and the larger salivatory duct of the sublingual gland.

Thomas Bartholin, elder

(1616–1680) Danish physician who gave the first description of the human lymphatic system, wrote the first Danish pharmacopoeia, and established the first Danish medical journal.

George Bartisch

(1535–1606) German ophthalmologist who wrote *Ophthalmodouleia. Das ist Augendienst*, which contains descriptions of eye surgery for cataract and strabismus, and used spectacles for visual correction.

John Rhea Barton

(1794–1871) American orthopedic surgeon, famous for being ambidextrous, who worked on arthroplasty and osteotomy, and performed subtrochanteric osteotomy of the femur for deformity.

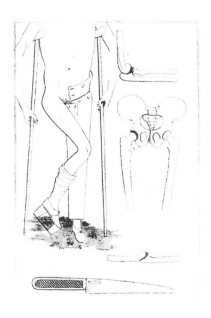

Ankylosis treatment

Agostino Maria Bassi

(1773–1856) Italian pioneer bacteriologist who demonstrated the fungal origin and contagiousness of silkworm disease, and proposed that micro-organisms were the cause of many diseases.

Henry Charlton Bastian

(1837–1915) British pioneer in clinical neurology who localized the centers in the brain controlling speech, and also studied the neurological basis of word blindness and word deafness.

Thomas Bateman

(1778–1821) British physician who wrote *Delineations of Cutaneous Diseases*, gave the first descriptions of molluscum contagiosum and ecthyma.

William Bateson

(1861–1926) Early British geneticist who translated and popularized Mendel's work, and showed the linked inheritance of some genes.

Julius Bauer

(1887–1979) Austrian endocrinologist who, in 1917, wrote *Constitution and Disease*, and was one of the first to suggest multiple hormones within a single gland.

Louis Bauer

(1814–1898) American orthopedic surgeon who wrote the first true US textbook on orthopedics, he also stressed rest and immobilisation for spinal injury.

Gaspard Laurent Bayle

(1774–1816) French physician who gave an original description of the tubercule in pulmonary and granular tuberculosis in his *Researches on Pulmonary Tuberculosis*.

Richard Bayley

(1745–1801) American physician who distinguished between diphtheria and putrid sore throat, organized the New York Dispensary, was health officer to the port, and studied yellow fever in the city.

Sir William M Bayliss

(1860–1924) British endocrinologist and gastro-enterologist who, in 1902 discovered secretin, wrote *Principles of General Physiology*, and *The Nature of Enzyme Action*.

Frank Ambrose Beach

(b 1911) American comparative psychologist and endocrinologist who studied hormonal regulation of reproductive behavior.

George Wells Beadle

(1903–1989) American geneticist and Nobel laureate who discovered that specific genes control production of specific enzymes.

Lionel Smith Beale

(1828–1906) British microscopist and histologist who used vital staining and discovered pyriform nerve ganglion cells.

William Beaumont

(1785–1853) American gastroenterologist who gave the first description of gastritis and the role of alcohol, studied digestion, describing it as a chemical process, and found hydrochloric acid in stomach juices.

Thomas Beddoes

(1760–1808) British physician who founded the Pneumatic Institute for treatment of diseases by inhalation therapy, and wrote *On Factitious Airs*.

Emil von Behring

(1854–1917) German pioneer immunologist who discovered antitoxins, developing serum therapy for tetanus and diphtheria using antitoxic sera. He was the first Nobel prizewinner in medicine or physiology (1901).

Martinus Willem Beijerinck

(1851–1931) Brilliant Dutch microbiologist who discovered the ultrafilterability of viruses and contributed to our understanding of the ecology of disease.

Georg von Békésy

(1899–1972) American physicist and physiologist who studied the ear and the mechanism of stimulation of the cochlea, and described how information is transmitted to the brain.

Vladimir M Bekhterev

(1857–1927) Russian neurologist who studied brain morphology, discovered the pontine superior vestibular nucleus, and described ankylosing spondylitis.

Sir Charles Bell

(1774–1842) British pioneer of neurophysiology who showed that nerves consist of separate fibers within a sheath and that the fibers convey either motor or sensory information in a single direction, described Bell's palsy due to paralysis of the 7th cranial nerve, and suggested a sitting position for amputation.

John Bell

(1763–1820) Brilliant British surgeon and anatomist who instigated ligation of aneurysms and wrote *The Anatomy of the Human Body*, *The Principles of Surgery and Discourses on the Nature and Cure of Wounds*.

Baruj Benacerraf

(b 1920) American–Venezuelan immunologist and Nobel laureate who was interested in hypersensitivity, discovered immune-response genes and clarified how cell-surface characteristics regulate responses to diseased cells and transplanted tissue.

Edouard van Beneden

(1846–1910) Belgian cytologist and embryologist who first revealed the constancy of chromosome numbers in cells of an organism, the halving of this number in germ cells and its restoration at fertilization.

Stanley R Benedict

(1884–1936) American hemalogist who devised the test for glycosuria, demonstrated the presence of

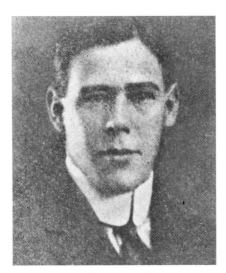

Stanley R Benedict

ammonia in urine was formed by the kidney, and measured metabolites in blood.

George Eli Bennett

(1885–1962) American orthopedic surgeon who worked through the polio epidemics of 1917 and 1946 and established the first respirator unit for bulbar palsy.

Seymour Benzer

(b 1921) American geneticist and member of the Phage Group who showed that changes in a gene led to changes in protein, introduced the term 'cistron' and identified 'hot spots' in DNA (sections particularly susceptible to mutation).

Paul Berg

(b 1926) American molecular biologist and Nobel laureate who worked with transfer RNAs and viruses, developed gene-splicing techniques, and was the first to transfer genes between cells from different mammal species.

Sune Karl Bergström

(b 1916) Swedish biochemist and Nobel prizewinner who studied metabolic pathways of cholesterol and prostaglandins.

Claude Bernard

(1813–1878) French physician and neurologist who, in 1855, differentiated between internal and external secretion of the liver, analyzed glandular extracts, studied carbohydrate metabolism and the sympathetic nervous system.

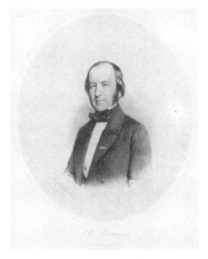

Claude Bernard

Paul Bert

(1833–1886) French physiologist and statesman who studied the effects of changes in atmospheric pressure, altitude, and composition of air on blood gases.

Arnold A Berthold

(1803–1861) German endocrinologist who showed that if a cock's testes were transplanted into its abdomen, its secondary sexual characteristics (including normal comb) were retained, proving that the testes produced a 'hormone'. This was a landmark discovery in endocrinology.

Jons Jacob Berzelius

(1779–1848) Swedish physician and chemist, a supporter of the atomic theory, he designed the modern system of chemical symbols, developed the electrochemical theory and studied the chemistry of urine.

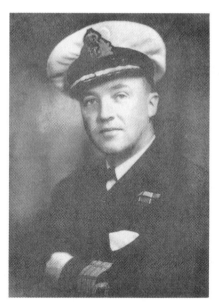

Charles H Best

Johann Ulric Bilguer

(1720–1796) German surgeon who wrote a monograph on amputation, and was the first to suggest conservative surgery of joints.

John Shaw Billings

(1838–1913) American military surgeon, planner of hospitals (including the Johns Hopkins) and founder of the world's greatest medical library, the National Library of Medicine.

Theodor Billroth

(1829–1894) German gastrologist and the founder of modern abdominal surgery who developed instruments and operations including partial gastrectomy, studied bacteria of wound fevers, and performed the first successful laryngectomy.

Charles H Best

(1899–1978) American endocrinologist and Nobel laureate in 1923 for discovery of insulin.

Marie FX Bichat

(1771–1802) French surgeon and pathologist who established the importance of physiology and pathology of tissues in disease. His book, *A Treatise on Membranes*, included the first accurate description of synovia.

Artur Biedl

(1869–1933) Austrian endocrinologist who, in 1910, published a two-volume book *Internal Secretion*, which is thought to be the first comprehensive treatise on ductless glands.

Henry J Bigelow

(1818–1890) American urologist and orthopedic surgeon who developed the Bigelow evacuator for crushing bladder stones and was the first to use the technique. He also did the first excision of a hip joint, treated hip dislocation, and introduced ether anesthesia.

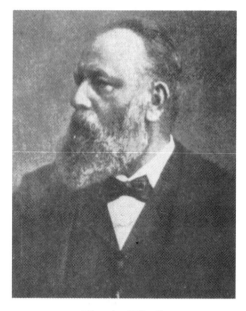

Theodor Billroth

Hildegard of Bingen

(1098–1179) German abbess, mystic and physician who wrote Physica, described plants used in medicine, and hygiene in pregnancy.

Golding Bird

(1814–1854) British physiologist and electrical therapist who wrote a monograph on urinary deposits, described oxaluria, and wrote *Elements of Natural Philosophy* (1839).

John Michael Bishop

(b 1936) American molecular biologist and Nobel laureate who discovered oncogenes, the normal cellular genes involved in growth and development and in which regulatory faults and lead to cancers.

Peter MF Bishop

(1904–1979) British endocrinologist and gynecologist who was a pioneer in female reproductive endocrinology, and investigated the actions of estrogen.

Joseph Black

(1728–1799) British scientist who discovered carbon dioxide by chemical analysis and in respiration, and also defined specific heat and latent heat.

Elizabeth Blackwell

(1821–1910) First woman to become a physician in America, established the New York Infirmary for Indigent Women and Children.

Alfred Blalock

(1899–1964) American heart surgeon who did the first 'blue baby' operation, studied surgical shock and its treatment by transfusion, and was the first to treat myasthenia gravis by removal of the thymus gland.

Konrad Emil Bloch

(b 1912) German-born American biochemist and Nobel laureate who elucidated cholesterol metabolism, opening up new approaches in the investigation of its role in atherosclerosis and heart disease.

Baruch Samuel Blumberg

(b 1925) American microbiologist and Nobel prizewinner who discovered the 'Australia antigen' and its relationship to hepatitis B, and developed a vaccine against HBV.

Johann Friedrich Blumenbach

(1752–1840) German scientist who was the founder of anthropology, and wrote *On the Native Varieties of the Human Race*, classifying racial characteristics based on skull shape, facial configuration, and skin color.

James Blundell

(1790–1877) British physiologist, obstetrician and one of the first to use blood transfusion. He developed pelvic surgery, differentiated between placenta previa and accidental hemorrhage, and performed vaginal hysterectomy for cervical cancer.

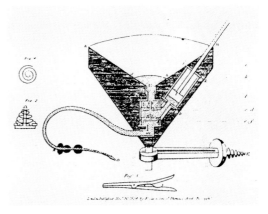

Blundell impellor

Ismar I Boas

(1858–1938) German gastrologist who developed a test meal to measure gastric secretion which he used in ulcer diagnosis, and also described occult blood in feces.

André Bocage

(1892–1953) Prolific French physician who studied skin diseases, dosage of staphylococcus toxoid in treatment of furunculosis, statistical errors in blood cell counting, developed a transfusion syringe and, most notably, was a pioneer of tomography.

Sir Walter Fred Bodmer

(b 1936) British geneticist who studied the HLA histocompatibility system that distinguishes self from non-self, and also contributed to understanding of cancer and population genetics.

Caesar Moeller Boeck

.(1845–1917) Norwegian dermatologist who described the skin lesion and histology of sarcoidosis and later showed the involvement of the spleen, liver, lungs and bone marrow.

Hermann Boerhaave

(1668–1738) Eminent Dutch chemist and physician who gave the first description of urea, wrote in 1708, *Medical Principles*, and described gout, dilatation of the heart, and spread of smallpox by contagion.

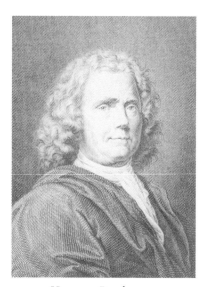

Hermann Boerhaave

Johann Bohn

(1640–1719) German physiologist who experimented on the decapitated frog and suggested that reflex action was entirely mechanical.

Theophile Bonet

(1620–1689) Swiss physician and anatomist who wrote a ground-breaking Guide to the *Practical*

Physician which classified diseases and symptoms with notes for diagnosis and treatment.

Amédée Bonnet

(1809–1858) French surgeon who wrote *Traité des maladies des articulations* on treatment for joint disease.

Jacobus Bontius

(1592–1631) Dutch physician to the East Indies Company who studied plants and diseases of this area, gave the first description of beriberi relating it to nutrition, and described cholera, yaws and dysentery.

Jules JBV Bordet

(1870–1961) Belgian bacteriologist and Nobel laureate who elucidated the mechanism of bacteriolysis and the two substances involved, discovered whooping cough bacillus and developed a vaccine from the endotoxin.

Théophile de Bordeu

(1722–1776) French physician and early endocrinologist who developed a theory of internal secretions, that each organ's emanations are useful and necessary to the body.

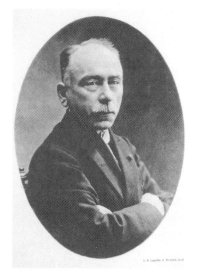

Jules Bordet

Bartolemmeo Borella

(1784–1854) Italian orthopedic surgeon who founded the first orthopedic institute in Italy (1823), and wrote *Cenni d'Ortopedia*.

Giovanni Alphonso Borelli

(1608–1679) Italian physician who wrote *De motu animalium*, applied mechanics and physical principles to the body, described locomotion, respiration, muscle action and digestion, and the neurogenic theory of heart action.

Teodorico Borgognoni

(c 1205–1298) Italian surgeon who contradicted Galenist theory, used mercury salves, and early anesthetics such as opium and mandragora.

Apollinaire Bouchardat

(1806–1886) French endocrinologist and the first to use polariscopic and chemical methods to detect diabetes, also developed diets and invented gluten-free bread.

Jean Baptiste Bouillaud

(1796–1881) French physician who was the first to show that aphasia was related to to a lesion in the anterior lobe of the brain, and described the association between rheumatic fever and heart disease.

Louyse Bourgeois

(1563–1636) French pioneer of scientific midwifery who wrote on female infertility, birth, and neonates.

Sauveur HV Bouvier

(1799–1877) French surgeon who wrote on bone deformities, the corset in history, and was the first to use the term 'locomotor apparatus'.

Theodor Heinrich Boveri

(1862–1915) German geneticist who studied fertilization. He described the centromere, and showed that each chromosome led to development of specific traits.

Daniel Bovet

(1907–1992) Italian biochemist and Nobel laureate who studied chemotherapeutics, discovered and developed the first antihistamine drugs, drugs for hypertension, and developed a synthetic derivative of curare used as a muscle relaxant in anesthetics.

Henry Pickering Bowditch

(1840–1911) American physiologist who worked on cardiac contraction, innervation of the heart, the knee-jerk reflex, and pioneered anthropometry in child growth.

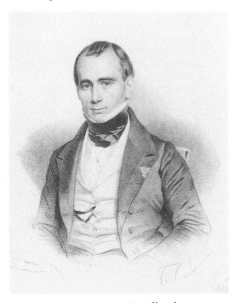

Jean Baptiste Bouillaud

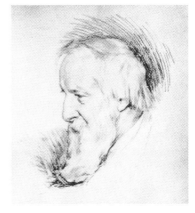

Henry Pickering Bowditch

Sir William Bowman

(1816–1892) British physician and ophthalmic surgeon who made significant discoveries concerning renal function, and described the ciliary muscle in his *Lectures on Operations on the Eye*.

William Clouser Boyd

(1903–1983) American immunochemist who studied antibody–antigen reactions, showed that blood groups are inherited, and distinguished humans into 13 distinct geographical races with different gene profiles.

Herbert Wayne Boyer

(b 1936) American pioneer in genetic engineering who developed cloning and hybridization, and showed how DNA of a plasmid could be joined to bacterial DNA.

Robert Boyle

(1627–1691) British natural philosopher and experimentalist who proved that air was needed for life and combustion, wrote a book of remedies including one for urinary calculi, and described hypothermia, and exophthalmic ophthalmoplegia.

Sir Byrom Bramwell

(1847–1931) British physician who, in 1888, suggested that obesity, polyuria and glucosuria in pituitary tumors may be caused by hypothalamic disturbance.

Lars G Branting

(1779–1881) Swedish orthopedic surgeon who developed a system of gymnastics in treatment which was adopted by many countries.

Antonio Musa Brassavola

(1500–1555) Italian physician who described over 200 kinds of syphilis, performed tracheotomy, wrote on purges, and introduced new drugs.

John Braxton Hicks

(1823–1897) British obstetrician and teacher who introduced a now obsolete method of fetal manipulation in placenta previa, the Braxton Hicks version, and described the painless contractions of later pregnancy.

Sydney Brenner

(b 1927) South African-born British molecular biologist who elucidated the nucleotide code for the 20 amino acids, and introduced the word 'codon' for a unit of three nucleotides that codes one amino acid.

Pierre Bretonneau

(1778–1862)
French physician who wrote monographs on typhoid and diphtheria (he named it in 1826), performed the first successful tracheotomy in croup, and suggested the germ theory of disease.

Richard Bright

(1789–1858) British physician and cardiologist who, in 1827, wrote *Reports of Medical Cases*, including a description of his eponymous disease, and, in 1832, wrote on pancreatic disease.

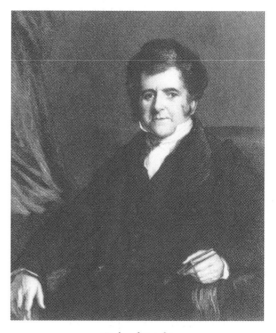

Richard Bright

Ralph Lawrence Brinster

(b 1932) American geneticist and Nobel laureate who was the first to introduce a human gene into the germline of a mouse, a technique now used to investigate the regulation of gene expression.

Pierre Brissot

(1478–1522) French physician who reformed bloodletting using free venesection near the lesion, but was banished for his work.

Roy John Britten

(b 1919) American molecular biologist who used nucleic acid hybridization to show that genomes of higher organisms contain more DNA than needed for a specific gene and its protein.

Paul Broca

(1824–1880) French surgeon and anthropologist who studied brain lesions and aphasia, and described the Broca gyrus, an area of the brain involved in motor speech.

Sir Benjamin C Brodie

(1783–1862) Eminent British surgeon and oncologist who wrote *On the pathology and surgery of diseases of the joints*, noted constitutional aspects of tuberculosis for which he advocated rest, and described Brodie tumor of the breast.

Detlev Wulf Bronk

(1887–1975) American neurophysiologist who isolated motor nerve fibers and studied their biophysical properties, studied the autonomic nervous system and the nervous control of cardiac function.

Lennox Ross Broster

(1889–1965) South African endocrinologist and surgeon who wrote The Adrenal Cortex and Intersexuality, in 1938.

François JV Broussais

(1772–1838) French physician who suggested that life depends on irritation or inflammation, particularly heat; that disease depends on local irritation and was, therefore, treated with extensive leeching and dietary deprivation.

John Brown

(1735–1788) British founder of the Brunonian theory of excitability of tissues, holding that disease was caused by excessive stimulation (treated by opium) or by insufficient stimulation (treated by alcohol).

John Ball Brown

(1784–1862) American orthopedic surgeon who did subcutaneous tenotomy of the Achilles tendon for club foot, tenotomy for torticollis, scoliosis and deformity.

Michael Stuart Brown

(b 1941) American biochemist and Nobel laureate who worked on cholesterol and hypocholesterolemia, showing that sufferers lacked a cell receptor for low-density lipoproteins, and found the code for this receptor.

Rachel Fuller Brown

(1898–1980) American biochemist who studied pneumonia and isolated nystatin, the first anti-fungal antibiotic.

Édouard Brown-Séquard

(1817–1894) French endocrinologist and neurologist who, in 1855, removed the adrenal glands, finding them to be essential to life, having a detoxicating effect. He also studied spinal cord lesions, including the effects of hemisection of the cord (Brown-Séquard syndrome).

Sir Thomas Browne

(1605–1682) British physician and writer who wrote Religio Medici, one of the greatest medical classics, *A Letter to a Friend*, *Vulgar Errors*, and *Christian Morals*.

Sir David Bruce

(1855–1931) Australian-born microbiologist who studied Brucella melitensis in cattle, the cause of brucellosis in man, and showed tsetse fly was the carrier of *Trypanosoma brucei*, responsible for sleeping sickness in humans.

Johann C Brunner

(1653–1727) Swiss physician who described glands in the duodenum, excised the pancreas and ligated the pancreatic duct in a dog and noted polydipsia and polyuria but made no association with diabetes.

Hieronymus Brunschwig

(1450–1533) German surgeon who wrote one of the first books describing the treatment of wounds, *Buch der Wund-Artzney*, regarded them as poisonous, and used amputation and cautery.

Sir Thomas Lauder Brunton

(1844–1916) Foremost British pharmacologist of his period who wrote *A Text Book of Pharmacology, Therapeutics and Materia Medica*, concentrated on understanding the mode of action of a drug and its application to restoration of health, and studied digitalis and amyl nitrite in heart disease.

Hans Buchner

(1850–1902) German microbiologist who studied gamma globulins, and showed that blood serum contains substances active against infections.

Gurdon Buck

(1807–1877) American orthopedic surgeon who treated femur fracture with adhesive strapping traction, much as used today.

Denis Parsons Burkitt

(1911–1993) Irish surgeon and nutritionalist who described Burkitt lymphoma in African children and related the low incidence of coronary heart disease and bowel cancer in Africans to their high fiber diet.

Sir Frank Macfarlane Burnet

(1899–1985) Australian microbiologist and Nobel laureate who developed a technique to culture viruses in living chick embryos, studied flu virus, graft rejection, and the production of specific antibodies on specialized white blood cells that bind invading antigens.

Adolf FJ Butenandt

(1903–1995) German endocrinologist and Nobel laureate for work on sex hormones, in particular his isolation of progesterone and the determination of its structure.

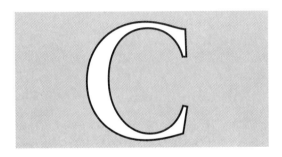

Richard Clark Cabot

(1868–1939) American hematologist who, in 1896, wrote *Clinical Examination of the Blood*, and described the fine blue-staining erythrocyte inclusions (Cabot rings) in megaloblastic anemia.

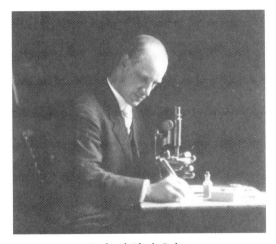

Richard Clark Cabot

Thomas Cadwalader

(1708–1779) American physician who provided an original description of West Indian dry gripes (lead poisoning from rum), another of softening of the bones, probably from osteitis fibrosa cystica generalisata, and was a pioneer of inoculation.

Hugh John Forster Cairns

(b 1922) British molecular biologist who showed that cancer develops from a single abnormal cell probably by DNA mutation but that further development depends on environment factors.

John Caius

(1510–1573) British physician and founder of the first medical college in England who wrote on the 'Sweatyng Sicknesse' – possibly plague, flu or rheumatic fever.

Albert Calmette

(1863–1933) French microbiologist who discovered anti-snakebite serum, described a diagnostic test for TB and developed inoculation with attenuated TB bacillus.

Jacques Calvé

(1875–1954) French orthopedic surgeon who described coxa plana, vertebral osteochondritis with collapse, and aspirated intraspinal abscesses in Pott disease.

Willis Campbell

(1880–1941) American orthopedic surgeon who wrote *Operative Orthopedics* (1939), and advocated interpositional arthroplasty.

Pieter Camper

(1722–1789) Dutch comparative anatomist, gynecologist and surgeon who was the first to propose symphysiotomy, described fascia and the olecranon bursa, wrote on shoe-induced deformities (1781) and vision.

Giambattista Canano

(1515–1579) Italian anatomist who wrote brilliantly and accurately on bones and muscles of the arm, using 26 illustrations produced by Girolamo da Carpi.

Walter B Cannon

(1871–1945) Brilliant American physiologist and neurologist who studied fight/fright responses, wrote *Bodily Changes in Pain, Hunger, Fear and Rage* in 1929, and introduced the term homeostasis in 1932.

Charles Robert Cantor

(b 1942) American molecular biologist who

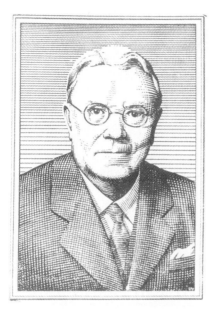

Walter B Cannon

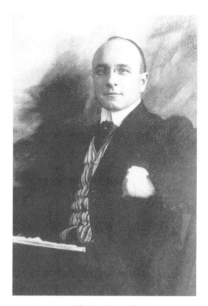

Alexis Carrel

developed pulse field gel electrophoresis for separating large DNA molecules, and is involved in the Human Genome Project.

Jerome Cardan

(1501–1576) French physician who was the first to suggest that the deaf could be taught using signs, and wrote *Metoposcopia* (1558), on physiognomy, with 800 illustrations of human faces.

Matthew Carey

(1760–1839) Irish-born American physician and publisher who gave an account of the yellow fever epidemic in Philadelphia.

William Benjamin Carpenter

(1813–1885) British neuropsychiatrist who worked on consciousness and unconsciousness, developing the theory of 'unconscious cerebration'.

Alexis Carrel

(1873–1944) French cardiologist who perfected leakproof vascular anastomizing techniques, used vein grafts, and was a Nobel laureate in 1912.

James Carroll

(1854–1907) American microbiologist who did research on yellow fever, establishing it as a virus – the first virus implicated in a human disease.

Robert Carswell

(1793–1857) British physician who wrote *Pathological Anatomy, Illustrations of the Elementary Forms of Disease* (1837), a classic atlas on gross pathology.

Henry Vandyke Carter

(1831–1897) British microbiologist who described mycetoma, leprosy, elephantiasis, and spirillosis.

Guilio Casseri

(1561–1616) Italian physician and early endocrinologist who described the thyroid as a single organ in two parts and without a duct.

Joseph Bienaimé Caventou

(1795–1877) French chemist who isolated chlorophyll, strychnine, quinine and cinchonine, veratrine, and caffeine.

Thomas Cech

(b 1947) American molecular biologist and Nobel laureate who discovered the function of RNA as a catalyst, showed that a protein-free precursor of ribosomal RNA mediates its own cleavage and splicing, identified ribozymes, and studied telomerase enzymes.

Aulus Cornelius Celsus

(c 25 BC–50 AD) Outstanding Greek physician and writer on medicine (De Medicina) who described anatomy, tuberculosis, scabies, cataracts, treatment of fractures, lithotomy, trephining, use of hemlock and opium, and many other aspects of medicine.

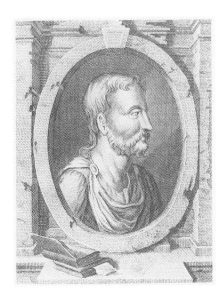

Aulus Cornelius Celsus

Andrea Cesalpino

(1519–1603) Italian botanist and physician who described the circulation, and theorized on systemic and pulmonary circulation.

Carlos Ribeiro Chagas

(1879–1934) Brazilian physician who studied malaria prevention and control, described Chagas disease, the causative organism *Trypanosomas cruzi* and the insect vector.

Sir Ernst Boris Chain

(1906–1979) American biochemist and Nobel laureate who identified a phospholipase in snake venom that paralyses the nervous system, determined the action of lysozyme on bacterial cell walls, and purified penicillin.

Nathaniel Chapman

(1780–1853) American physician, obstetrician and first president of the American Medical Association, who also established the first postgraduate medical school, and wrote an outstanding treatise for the period, *Elements of Therapeutics and Materia Medica.*

Jean Martin Charcot

(1825–1893) Renowned French physician and surgeon who was the first professor of neurology, distinguished gout from rheumatoid arthritis, rheumatoid from osteoarthritis, described muscular atrophy, studied multiple sclerosis, spastic paralysis and hysteria.

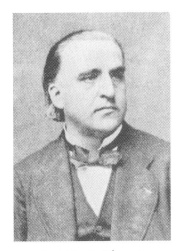

Jean Martin Charcot

Erwin Chargaff

(b 1905) American biochemist who studied bacterial lipids, the paired composition of DNA bases, and showed that DNA was specific within a species.

Sir John Charnley

(1911–1982) British orthopedic surgeon and a pioneer of compression arthrodesis and low-friction hip arthroplasty.

Gaspard A Chatin

(1813–1901) French endocrinologist who showed that cretinism was directly related to iodine deficiency, and calculated the amount needed.

Guy de Chauliac

(c 1300–1368) Great French physician and surgeon who wrote *Chirugia Magna and Parva*, recommended removal of the thyroid for goiter, described fracture treatment with traction and use of a special bed, used narcotics in surgery, operated on hernia, cataract and cancer, and performed dentistry.

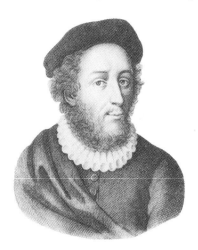

Guy de Chauliac

Chu Chen-Heng

(c 1500) Chinese physician who wrote on the use of the placenta and urine extracts in infertility and dysmenorrhea.

William Cheselden

(1688–1752) British surgeon who carried out tenotomy for torticollis, performed iridectomy, lithotomy (in 54 seconds!), and wrote *Anatomy of the Human Body*, and Osteographia.

John Cheyne

(1777–1836) Irish physician who described hydrocephalus (1808), hypochondriasis ('the English malady'), and Cheyne-Stokes respiration (1818).

Russell Henry Chittenden

(1856–1943) American biochemist who studied toxicology and human nutritional requirements, and suggested that over-rich protein diets may cause health problems.

Albert Claude

(1899–1983) Belgian cell biologist and Nobel laureate in 1974 who pioneered the process of cell fractionation using a high-powered centrifuge, and the use of the electron microscope in cell biology

Mather Cleveland

(1889–1979) American orthopedic surgeon who was a pioneer in treatment of skeletal tuberculosis.

Alessandro Codivilla

(1861–1912) Italian orthopedic surgeon who wrote on tendon transplantation and redistribution of muscle power around a joint, and used it in spastic paralysis.

Ernest A Codman

(1869–1940) American orthopedic surgeon and an early user of X-rays who wrote on bone tumors, and described chondroblastoma.

Seymour Stanley Cohen

(b 1917) American biochemist who isolated thromboplastin from lung tissue, demonstrated its importance in clotting, that it was a phospholipo-protein, and studied T phage activation and inactivation using UV light.

Stanley Cohen

(b 1922) American cell biologist and Nobel laureate in 1986 who isolated nerve growth factors from *in vitro* tissue culture.

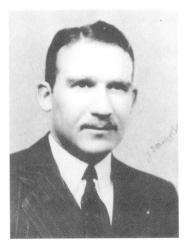

Stanley Cohen

Julius F Cohnheim

(1839–1884) German experimental pathologist who first described the microscopic features of inflammation, proved that TB was an infectious disease, studied coronary artery obstruction and developed frozen section and new staining techniques.

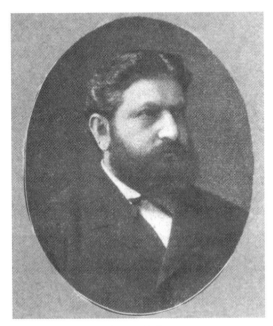

Julius Cohnheim

Volcher Coiter

(1534–1590) Italian physician who showed that the ovary is not the source of sperm, described the corpus luteum, growth and formation of bones, and the muscles of the nose and eyelids.

Abraham Colles

(1773–1843) Irish physician and surgeon remembered for Colles fracture of the radius, he was the first to tie the right subclavian artery, and described Colles fascia, a membraneous layer of the perineum.

James B Collip

(1892–1965) Canadian biochemist who described several placental and anterior pituitary hormones, worked on the isolation of insulin and discovered the active principal of the parathyroid gland in 1925.

Matteo Realdo Colombo

(1516–1559) Italian anatomist who gave one of the earliest descriptions of pulmonary circulation, wrote *De re anatomica*, showed that pulmonary veins contain blood made 'spiritous' by lungs, and observed that the thyroid in the female is larger than in the male.

Robin RA Coombs

(b 1921) British immunologist who developed a test for red cell antibodies which is used in blood transfusion matching and diagnosis of anemia.

Sir Astley Paston Cooper

(1768–1841) British surgeon and a pioneer in vascular and experimental surgery, wrote on the testis, the thymus, and breast disease, and treated compound fractures by total immobilisation. He was the first surgeon to treat aneurysm by tying the abdominal aorta.

Valerius Cordus

(1515–1544) German physician who wrote *Pharmacorum Conficiendorum Ratio* (1546) the first real pharmacopoeia, and discovered sulfuric ether.

Carl Ferdinand Cori

(1896–1984) American biochemist and Nobel laureate who isolated glucose-1-phosphate from muscle, glycogen phosphorylase and its prosthetic group adenylic acid.

Gerty Theresa Cori (nee Houssay)

(1896–1957) American biochemist and Nobel laureate who studied carbohydrate metabolism, glycogen breakdown, and the effects of hormones and tumors on its pathway.

George W Corner

(1889–1981) American endocrinologist who developed our understanding of the ovulatory cycle, particularly the role of progesterone.

Andre-Victor Cornil

(1837–1908) French physician and organ pathologist who wrote on pathology of the kidneys, studied juvenile rheumatoid arthritis, and showed sodium urate to be presenting joints in gout.

Sir Dominic J Corrigan

(1802–1880) Irish physician who described famine fever in 1847, wrote on aortitis and mitral stenosis and gave an original description of aortic insufficiency and the waterhammer pulse, typical of aortic regurgitation.

Jean N Corvisart

(1755–1821) French cardiologist who established percussion in diagnosis of heart disease, described arrhythmias and mitral stenosis, and distinguished cardiac hypertrophy from dilatation.

Domenico Cotugno

(1736–1822) Italian physician, anatomist and surgeon who studied cerebrospinal fluid, distinguished arthritic sciatica from nervous sciatica, and described the anatomy of the inner ear.

André Frédéric Cournand

(1895–1988) Nobel laureate and American pioneer in cardiac catheterization, threading a catheter

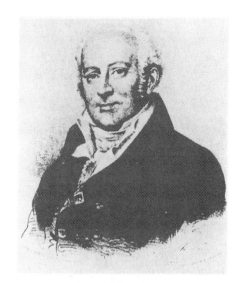

Jean N Corvisart

through an arm or leg vein into the right atrium of the heart, so enabling him to study conditions in the heart without using surgery.

Ludwig G Courvoisier

(1843–1918) Swiss surgeon and a pioneer in biliary tract surgery and gallbladder disease, remembered for his diagnostic Law and sign, who used cholecystectomy in treatment.

William Cowper

(1666–1709) British physician who wrote *The Anatomy of Human Bodies*, and described the bulbourethral glands.

Carl SF Crede

(1819–1892) German gynecologist and obstetrician who advocated gentle manipulation for expulsion of the placenta and introduced silver nitrate instillation for prevention of ophthalmia neonatorum.

Francis Harry Compton Crick

(b 1916) British biochemist and Nobel laureate who elucidated the structure of DNA as a double helix of two chains of nucleotide bases wound around a common axis in opposite directions.

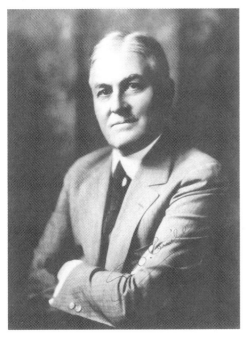

George W Crile

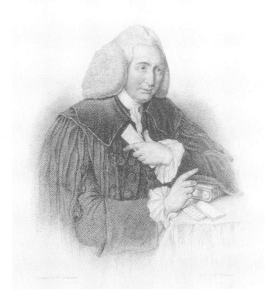

William Cullen

George W Crile

(1864–1943) American physiologist and surgeon who studied surgical shock, developed nerve block anesthesia, and latterly worked on surgery of the thyroid.

William Croone

(1633–1684) British physician who wrote on muscular physiology and embryology of the chick, and endowed the Croonian lectures.

William C Cruikshank

(1745–180) British physician who studied reunion and regeneration of divided nerves, passage of the ovum through the Fallopian tubes, perspiration and loss of carbon dioxide through the skin.

Jean Cruveilhier

(1791–1874) French pathologist who gave early descriptions of gastric ulcer, pyloric stenosis, disseminated sclerosis, and congenital cirrhosis.

William Cullen

(1710–1790) British physician and nosologist who gave the first lectures in the vernacular, developed hydrotherapy, and divided disease into fevers, neuroses, cachexias and local disorders.

Nicholas Culpeper

(1616–1654) British physician and apothecary who wrote and translated a prodigious number of treatises into English for use by the general public, including a notable herbal.

Marie Curie

(1867–1936) French physicist who discovered polonium and radium, developed X-radiography, and was awarded Nobel Prizes for Physics (1903) and Chemistry (1911).

Pierre Curie

(1859–1906) French physicist and Nobel laureate who discovered piezoelectricity and developed an electrometer to measure it, and showed rays emitted by radium to contain positive, negative and neutral particles.

Thomas Blizard Curling

(1811–1888) British surgeon who studied tetanus, duodenal ulcers associated with burns, wrote a book on the rectum and testes, and a paper on thyroid and poor cerebral development in which he suggested that absence of the thyroid was responsible for the systemic symptoms.

James Currie

(1756–1805) British physician who used cold baths in treatment of typhoid and other febrile diseases, and checked his results with a thermometer.

Harvey Williams Cushing

(1869–1939) American neurosurgeon who studied pituitary tumors and over-secretion by the adrenal cortex.

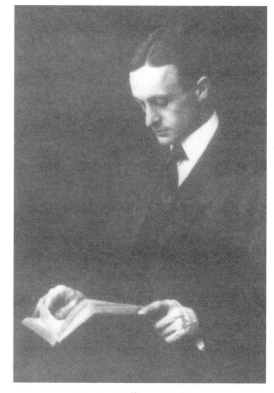

Harvey Williams Cushing

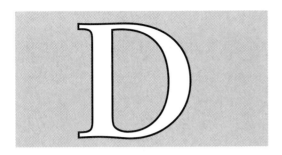

Sir Henry H Dale

(1875–1968) British physiologist and Nobel laureate for work on the chemical transmission of nerve impulses, who described acetylcholine and norepinephrine.

John C Dalton Jr.

(1825–1889) First professor of physiology in America who wrote the first major text on the subject in the US and a further text for household use.

Carl Peter Henrik Dam

(1895–1976) Danish-born American biochemist and Nobel laureate who discovered vitamin K, the anti-hemorrhagic vitamin essential for synthesis of prothrombin, while researching cholesterol metabolism.

Walter Dandy

(1886–1946) American neurosurgeon who introduced pneumoencephalography in diagnosis of tumors, and studied hydrocephalus and cerebro-spinal fluid.

James Frederic Danielli

(1911–1984) British–American cell physiologist and Nobel Laureate who studied cell membrane structure and transport of molecules across membranes, and proposed that the membrane is a 'sandwich' of proteins with lipids in the middle.

Cyril Dean Darlington

(1903–1981) British cytologist and geneticist who developed seven theories and proposed 60 genetic terms, and suggested that chromosomes were subject to selection and evolution.

Raymond Arthur Dart

(1893–1988) Australian-born South African anatomist who described and named a possible human ancestor, *Australopithecus africanus*, and suggested that bipedalism preceded brain expansion.

Jean Baptiste Gabriel Dausset

(b 1916) French immunologist and Nobel laureate who studied transfusion and antibody response, tissue rejection, and developed tissue typing.

Casimir Joseph Davaine

(1812–1882) French physician and microbiologist who was the first to identify the anthrax bacillus, studied parasitic worms, and advocated the germ theory of disease.

Eric Harris Davidson

(b 1937) American molecular biologist who elucidated genome organization and gene regulation, and found 'junk' DNA whose function remains unknown.

Jacques Daviel

(1696–1762) French physician who did the first extraction of the lens for cataract, and wrote a treatise on it.

Leonardo Da Vinci

(1452–1519) Italian and the greatest artist and scientist of the Renaissance, who said that glands existed to close the gaps where there were no muscles, that the thyroid separated the trachea from the clavicle, and studied skeletal movement and muscle structure in relation to function.

Henry G Davis

(1806–1896) American orthopedic surgeon and pioneer in sanatoria for tuberculosis, who did open evacuation of suppurative arthritis, washing out with chlorine and water.

Hugh Davson

(b 1909) British physiologist who studied membrane permeability (with Danielli), the nature of fluids in the eye in relation to glaucoma, and spinal fluids.

Humphry Davy

(1778–1829) British scientist who studied gases and discovered the anesthetic properties of nitrous oxide (laughing gas).

Felix Vicq d'Azyr

(1748–1794) French neurologist and anatomist who studied flexor and extensor muscles, morphology of brain, and the vocal cords. He was the greatest comparative anatomist of the period,the first to section the brain horizontally and the first to identify cerebral convolutions, basal ganglia and deep gray nuclei.

Christian René De Duve

(b 1917) Belgian biochemist and Nobel laureate who discovered lysosomes and peroxisomes in the cell while studying carbohydrate metabolism, and showed that malfunction of lysosomes causes cystinosis and other metabolic diseases.

Johann Deisenhofer

(b 1943) American biochemist and Nobel prizewinner who studied X-ray crystallography of biological macromolecules, immunoglobulin structure, identified biomolecule receptor and effector sites, and studied energetics of protein-DNA interactions.

Augusta Klumpke Dejerine

(1859–1927) American neurologist who, with her husband, discovered Dejerine-Klumpke paralysis, which results from injury to the lower brachial plexus, and wrote on lead palsy.

Joseph Dejerine

(1849–1917) French neurologist who studied motor neurone disease, tabes dorsalis, muscular dystrophy, the effects of nutritional deficiency, and aphasia.

Max Delbrück

(1906–1981) German-born American biophysicist and Nobel laureate who studied genetics of the phage virus, showed that viruses can exchange genetic material to create new viruses, and set up the Phage Group.

Jacques M Delpech

(1777–1832) French surgeon who invented subcutaneous Achilles tenotomy, wrote *De l'orthomorphie*, and had a gymnasium for patients in his clinic.

Pierre Joseph Desault

(1744–1795) French surgeon and the founder of *Journal de Chirurgie*, who developed techniques for ligating blood vessels in aneurysms.

René Descartes

(1596–1650) French physician, philosopher, mathematician and natural scientist who distinguished between sensory and motor nerves, studied the functioning of the eye and heart muscle action, and wrote *Discours de la methode*, on how to do research.

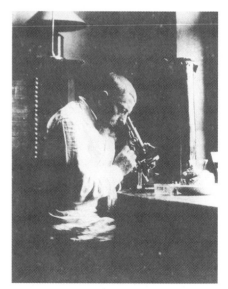

Joseph Dejerine

William Ludwig Detmold

(1808–1894) American orthopedic surgeon who did the first subcutaneous tenotomy in the US.

Hendrik van Deventer

(1651–1724) Dutch obstetrician, the father of modern midwifery, and an orthopedic surgeon, who wrote *Novum Lumen*, giving the first accurate description of the pelvis and its deformities, spinal deformities, creating appliances for them, and treated Kristian V's children for rickets deformities.

Hugo Marie De Vries

(1848–1935) Dutch geneticist who studied heredity in plants, developed Mendelian genetics and evolutionary and mutation theories, and discovered the plasmalemma and the phenomenon of plasmolysis.

Felix D'Hérelle

(1873–1949) French–Canadian bacteriologist and one of the founders of molecular biology, who discovered the bacteriophage in 1915, and tried to use it therapeutically (but unsuccessfully).

Johann F Dieffenbach

(1792–1847) German surgeon who was a pioneer in transplant surgery, worked on blood transfusion and plastic surgery and was the first to use subcutaneous drilling and insertion of ivory pegs for pseudoarthrosis.

Pedanus Dioscorides

(c AD 40–90) Greek physician who collected plants and produced a *Materia Medica* (he introduced this term) which described the use of opium, cures for worms, and the use of colchicum for arthritis and gout.

Carl Djerassi

(b 1923) American pioneer of oral contraceptives who studied the chemistry of natural products using mass spectroscopy and circular dichroism.

Matthew Dobson

(1735–1784) British physician who wrote *Experiments and Observations on the Urine in Diabetes*, showed that sugar was present in urine and blood, and described hyperglycemia.

Theodosius Dobzhansky

(1900–1975) American geneticist who showed there to be a large degree of genetic variability in the population including many potentially lethal recessive genes, wrote *Genetics and the Origin of Species, and Heredity, Race and Society*.

Sir Edward Charles Dodds

(1899–1973) British endocrinologist and biochemist who isolated many hormones, and developed the synthetic hormones stilboestrol, and hexestrol.

Peter C Doherty

(b 1940) Australian immunologist and Nobel prizewinner who elucidated the mechanism of recognition by the immune system (T lymphocytes) of virus-infected cells. He showed that a signal from the virus on the cell surface and another from the host cell MHC must be recognized before a host cell is destroyed.

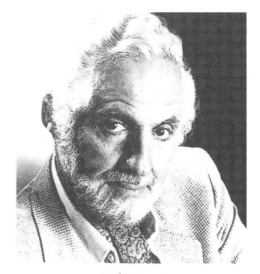

Carl Djerassi

29

Edward A Doisy

(1893–1986) American biochemist and Nobel laureate for work on vitamin K structure, who studied the hormonal mechanism of the estrous cycle and the chemical actions of insulin on the blood.

Gerhard Johannes Paul Domagk

(1895–1964) German biochemist and Nobel prizewinner who developed the combination of azo dye and prontosil which was converted to sulfanilamide in the body,for treatment of infections, thus opening up a new era of chemotherapy.

Franciscus Cornelis Donders

(1818–1889) Dutch ophthalmologist who improved the efficiency of spectacles with the introduction of prismatic and cylindrical lenses, and wrote on eye physiology.

Paul Mead Doty

(b 1920) American molecular biologist who discovered DNA renaturation so establishing the possibility of DNA hybridization.

Thomas Dover

(1660–1742) British physician and swashbuckler who invented the Dover Powder, a compound of ipecacuanha, opium, licorice, saltpetre and tartar vitroleus, for treatment of gout and gouty arthritis, cough and other pains.

Daniel Drake

(1785–1852) American physician who wrote *A Systematic Treatise, Historical, Etiological, and A Practical, on the Principal Diseases of the Interior Valleys of North America, as They Appear in the Caucasian, African, Indian, and Esquimaux Varieties of Its Population* in two volumes!

Hans Adolf Eduard Driesch

(1867–1941) German physiologist who was the first to provide evidence against the preformation theory of embryology with his work on the sea urchin.

Emil Heinrich Du Bois-Reymond

(1818–1896) German physiologist who discovered that nerves transmit electrical currents and also detected impulse in individual muscle fibers.

René Jules Dubos

(1901–1982) American bacteriologist who, in 1939, isolated tyrothricin from *Bacillus brevis*, which became the first commercially produced antibiotic.

Guillaume A Duchenne

(1806–1875) Distinguished French physician and neurologist who described many neuromuscular diseases including pseudohypertrophic muscular atrophy, and developed a machine for electrical stimulation of nerves.

Renato Dulbecco

(b 1914) Italian–American virologist who showed that certain viruses can transform cells into a cancerous state, making them grow continuously.

Guillaume Dupuytren

(1777–1835) French surgeon and pathologist who wrote on congenital dislocation of the hip, described a fracture of the fibula complicated by dislocation of the ankle joint, and his eponymous contracture of the palmar fascia, callus formation, and subungual exostosis.

Henri Dutrochet

(1776–1847) French physician who suggested that cellular respiration was the same in plants and animals and that all life processes could be explained in physicochemical terms.

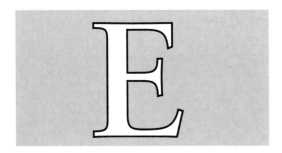

Sir John C Eccles

(1903–1997) Australian neurophysiologist and Nobel laureate who studied the mechanism of interneuronal communication and synapses, and kidney and heart function.

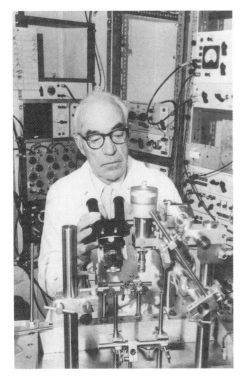

John Eccles

Constantin von Economo

(1876–1931) Austrian neurologist who identified and characterized epidemic encephalitis in 1918 and showed it was caused by a submicroscopic virus.

Gerald Maurice Edelman

(b 1929) American molecular biologist and Nobel laureate who purified the light chain of a human myeloma, analyzing its complete amino acid sequence, and studied antibody structure and subunit interactions.

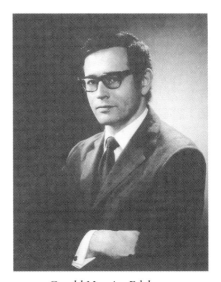

Gerald Maurice Edelman

Robert Geoffrey Edwards

(b 1925) British pioneer in reproductive physiology, fertility, infertility and the process of conception, who developed in vitro fertilization.

Antonio Egas Moniz

(1874–1955) Portuguese neurosurgeon and Nobel laureate in 1949, who introduced cerebral angiography for the localization of intracranial tumors, and performed prefrontal lobotomy for schizophrenia and other mental illness.

Paul Ehrlich

(1854–1915) German Nobel laureate, pioneer in chemotherapy and hematology who developed specific stains for white blood cells, introduced the differential blood cell count, and developed the side-chain theory of immunology, and synthesized salvarsan for the treatment of syphilis.

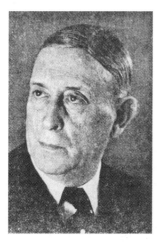

Antonio Egas Moniz

Christiaan Eijkman

(1858–1930) Dutch physician and Nobel prize-winner who proposed the concept of 'essential food factors'. He studied beriberi and showed it to be a deficiency disease (now known to be a deficiency of vitamin A).

Willem Einthoven

(1860–1927) Dutch physiologist and Nobel laureate who invented the string galvanometer, and was made a Nobel laureate for his work on electrocardiography.

Gertrude B Elion

(b 1918) American biochemist and Nobel laureate in 1988 who synthesized anti-cancer and antimalarial drugs, and acyclovir which is used in AIDS treatment.

Conrad Arnold Elvehjem

(1901–1962) American biochemist who showed that trace elements are necessary in nutrition and studied the deficiency disease pellagra, showing that liver extract could cure it.

Gladys Anderson Emerson

(b 1903) American biochemist who first isolated vitamin E, studied the role of B vitamins in disease and investigated possible dietary causes of cancer.

John Franklin Enders

(1897–1985) American microbiologist and Nobel laureate who studied antibodies to the mumps virus, established a polio research laboratory, cultured polio virus in human tissue culture, and developed a measles vaccine.

Rufus of Ephesus

(98–117) Greek physician who wrote *On the Interrogation of the Patient*, gave the earliest description of the thymus, wrote on the eye, liver, heart and pulse, gout, bubonic plague and erysipelas.

Sir Michael Anthony Epstein

(b 1921) British oncologist and microbiologist who discovered Epstein-Barr virus, the first virus shown to be associated with cancers in humans, and also associated with infectious mononucleosis.

Erasistratus of Ceos

(300–250 BC) Early Greek anatomist who rejected the notion of spirits, suggested that digestion was

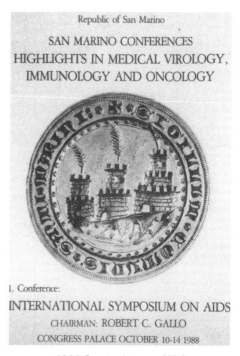

1988 Symposium on AIDS

involved in peristaltic motion of gastric muscles, studied the brain and cardiovascular system, noted differences between sensory and motor nerves and thought nerves were hollow tubes filled with fluids containing the 'nervous spirit'.

Desiderius Erasmus

(1466–1536) Dutch scholar and humanist who suggested the relationship between infection and 'foul air', and wrote *In Praise of the Healing Arts*.

Wilhelm Erb

(1840–1921) German neurologist who developed the use of the reflex hammer, popularized electro-diagnosis, described myasthenia gravis, brachial palsy, syphilitic spinal paralysis, and classified the myopathies.

Jakob Erdheim

(1874–1937) Austrian endocrinologist who studied pituitary tumors, craniopharyngiomas, dwarfism, acromegaly, and bone disorders.

Joseph Erlanger

(1874–1965) American neurophysiologist and Nobel laureate who studied electrophysiology of nerve activity and related speed of transmission to fiber thickness.

Dominique Esquirol

(1772–1840) French physician, one of the founders of modern psychiatry, who experimented with techniques for the control of epilepsy, and reformed the treatment of the insane.

Charles Estienne

(d 1564) French physician who was the first to call valves in veins apophyses membranarum, and gave the first description of syringomyelia.

Ulf von Euler

(1905–1983) Swedish pharmacologist and Nobel Laureate in 1970, who identified the transmitter of the sympathetic nervous system, norepinephrine, and discovered prostaglandins.

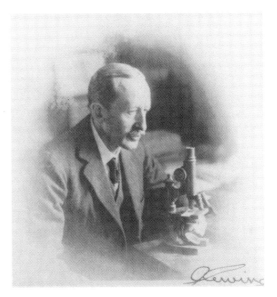

James Ewing

Hans KAS von Euler-Chelpin

(1873–1964) Swedish biochemist and Nobel prizewinner who studied the peptidases, saccharases and zymase showing that it was activated by vitamins A and B.

Bartolemmeo Eustachio

(1520–1574) Italian morphologist and anatomist who described auditory tubes, cochlea, thoracic duct, optic nerve, heart, suprarenal glands, uterus, and the sympathetic nervous system. He studied the kidney and suggested that urine flowed through canaliculi towards the calyces.

James Ewing

(1866–1943) American oncologist and first professor of pathology at Cornell who wrote an important reference work on diagnosis and treatment of neoplastic diseases in 1919, and described Ewing sarcoma of the bone.

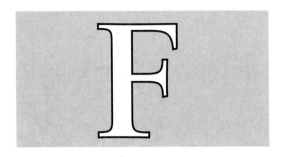

Gabriele Falloppio

(1523–1562) Great Italian anatomist who described the tubes named after him, the round ligaments, the cochlea and labyrinth of the ear, and differentiated mucosa, submucosa and muscle coats of viscera.

Arthur Fallot

(1850–1911) French cardiologist remembered for describing a congenital abnormality of the heart and great vessels, Fallot tetralogy.

Wilhelm Falta

(1875–1950) Austrian endocrinologist who studied endocrine and metabolic disorders, including diabetes mellitus, and wrote *The Diseases of the Bloodglands*.

Juan Farrill

(1902–1973) Mexican orthopedic surgeon who introduced skeletal traction and fixation, myelography for diagnozing disc lesions, and arteriography for bone tumor diagnosis.

Sir Joseph Fayrer

(1824–1907) British physician who wrote *The Thanatophidia of India*, which describes experiments using venoms.

Honor Bridget Fell

(1900–1986) British cell biologist who studied organ culture methods, using them to study the physiological effects of vitamins and hormones, and later investigated the pathogenesis of arthritis.

Otfried O Fellner

(b 1873) German endocrinologist and gynecologist who studied reproductive endocrinology, hormonal contraception, and placental function.

Gary Felsenfeld

(b 1929) American molecular biologist who developed DNA footprinting for studying the association between regulatory protein molecules and chromatin in the regulation of globin genes.

Samuel Fenwick

(1821–1902) British gastroenterologist who described atrophic gastritis, and wrote *Morbid States of the Stomach and Duodenum* in 1865.

Sir William Fergusson

(1808–1877) British surgeon remembered for his conservative and preservative surgical methods operations for hare lip and cleft palate, excision of the head of the femur and removal of the knee joint, and operations for vesical calculus.

Jean Fernel

(1497–1588) Remarkable French physician who wrote *Universa Medicina* covering pathology, physiology and therapeutics, who described aneurysms in the thoracic and abdominal cavities.

Sir David Ferrier

(1843–1928) British neurologist who studied the cerebral cortex in surgical and electro-stimulation experiments on animals, and published *The Functions of the Brain* in 1876.

Stubbins H Ffirth

(1784–1820) American epidemiologist who made an important study of yellow fever based on extensive animal and self-experimentation, and showed that it could not be transmitted through ingestion, injection or inhalation describing it a 'noncontagious', contrary to current opinion.

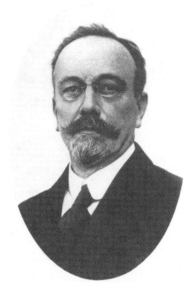

Johannes AG Fibiger

Johannes AG Fibiger

(1867–1928) Danish pathologist and Nobel laureate in 1926 who induced squamous cell carcinoma in the stomach of rats by feeding them on cockroaches infected by the nematode parasite *Spiroptera neoplastica*, stimulating much further cancer research.

Adolph Eugen Fick

(1829–1901) Exemplary German physiologist who studied the blind spot in the eye, calculated cardiac output, and developed a law of diffusion of liquids in relation to concentration gradient.

Carlos Juan Finlay

(1833–1915) Cuban microbiologist who studied the spread of yellow fever and showed it to be spread by mosquitoes, and then experimented on the production of immunity, allowing infected mosquitoes to bite healthy subjects.

Niels Ryberg Finsen

(1860–1904) Danish physician and Nobel laureate who studied effects of light in disease. He showed that blue and UV light caused inflammation but that red and infrared light were therapeutic in patients with smallpox, and used UV light to treat lupus vulgaris.

Emil Fischer

(1852–1919) Brilliant German biochemist and Nobel Laureate who discovered phenylhydrazine, synthesized aldehydes, ketones, purines, identified amino acids and uric acid, recognizing the latter's importance in gout.

Sir Ronald Aylmer Fisher

(1890–1962) British statistician and geneticist who wrote *Statistical Methods for Research Workers*, and elucidated the rhesus factor in his work on the genetics of human blood groups.

Reginald H Fitz

(1843–1913) British gastrologist who wrote a classic text on perforated appendix in 1886, was one of the first to advocate surgical treatment for acute appendicitis, and described acute pancreatitis.

Richard Anthony Flavell

(b 1945) British biochemist who studied structure and expression of human globin genes, found defects responsible for thalassemias involving total deletion of a gene for a specific globin, and developed gene therapy for such anemias.

Sir Alexander Fleming

(1881–1955) British bacteriologist and Nobel laureate who discovered the first antibiotic, penicilli,n in 1928, and pioneered anti-typhoid vaccination, and the use of salvarsan against syphilis.

Simon Flexner

(1863–1946) American microbiologist who isolated the dysentery bacillus, helped determine the cause of polio, and developed a serum for cerebrospinal meningitis.

Austin Flint Sr

(1812–1886) American cardiologist who wrote *On Cardiac Murmurs* in 1862, describing patho-

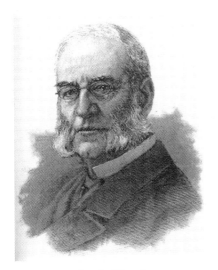

Austin Flint Sr

physiological symptoms, and gave the first description of the presystolic murmur of aortic incompetence.

Howard Walter Florey

(1898–1968) Australian pathologist and Nobel laureate who synthesized many antibiotics, in particular, penicillin, supervising its clinical trials in the USA.

Pierre Jean Marie Flourens

(1794–1867) French physiologist who studied the central nervous system, showed that respiration was controlled by the medulla oblongata, that vision depended on the integrity of the cerebral cortex, and that coordination of movement was controlled by the cerebellum.

Sir John Floyer

(1649–1734) British physician who measured pulse rate using a specially invented 'Physician's' Pulse Watch, making many observations on pulse frequency, and advocated cold baths.

Otto KO Folin

(1867–1934) Swedish-born American biochemist who developed colorimetric micromethods for urine and blood analysis, and showed that proteins were broken down into amino acids before they were absorbed.

Karl August Folkers

(b 1906) American biochemist who isolated cyanocobalamin, vitamin B12, from liver, mevalonic acid from a byproduct of yeast, and elucidated the structure of thyrotrophin-releasing hormone.

Felice Fontana

(1730–1803) French physician who studied effects of viper venom and stimulation of the cerebral cortex with electricity, and was the first to clearly visualize cell nuclei.

Edmund Brisco Ford

(1901–1988) British geneticist who showed that expression of a trait in successive generations was under genetic control, and that maintenance of different inherited forms of a character in a population can result from natural selection.

Werner Forssmann

(1904–1979) German surgeon who pioneered cardiac catheterization in his search for a method of injecting drugs directly into the heart, trying it first on himself.

Sir Michael Forster

(1836–1907) British cardiologist who studied the mechanism of heartbeat and intrinsic rhythmicity and neural regulation.

John Fothergill

(1712–1780) British physician who wrote *An Account of the Sore Throat Attended with Ulcers: A Disease Which Hath of Late Years Appeared in This City, and the Parts Adjacent*, gave original descriptions of diphtheria, and described facial neuralgia.

Girolamo Fracastorio

(c 1478–1553) Italian physician, physicist, astronomer and pathologist who made the first reference to magnetic poles of the Earth, studied and named venereal diseases, including syphilis, described foot-and-mouth infection, and provided an original description of typhus fever.

Heinz Fraenkel-Conrat

(b 1910) American biochemist who reconstituted the tobacco mosaic virus from the inactive protein and nucleic acids, thus showing it to be a basic unit in molecular biology, and developed sequencing and modification of RNA.

Johann Peter Frank

(1745–1821) German founder of preventative medicine and public hygiene who wrote *System of a Complete Medical Police*, and distinguished diabetes insipidus from diabetes mellitus.

Benjamin Franklin

(1706–1790) American scientist, inventor and statesman who invented bifocal lenses, a flexible catheter, and wrote on use of electricity in paralysis, gout, infective nature of colds, and infant death rate.

Pierre Franco

(1500–1561) French surgeon who operated for hernia, stone, cataract, and did the first suprapubic cystotomy.

John Freke

(1688–1756) British surgeon and first curator of the pathological museum of St Bartholomew's Hospital, who advocated drainage of the pleural cavity in empyema as soon as the breath sounds altered.

Friedrich Theodor von Frerichs

(1819–1885) German pathologist and founder of the science of experimental patholgy, whose work laid the foundations for modern clinical medicine. His studies of the biochemistry of diseased organs improved diagnosis and treatment of liver diseases and diabetes.

Sigmund Freud

(1856–1939) Austrian psychiatrist and neurologist who developed psychoanalysis, used hypnosis to study the unconscious, and developed the concepts of id, ego and superego.

Alfred Fröhlich

(1871–1953) Austrian neurologist who described Fröhlich syndrome in 1901, adiposogenital dystrophy, associated with a tumor of the pituitary.

Leonhard Fuchs

(1501–1566) German physician and botanist who wrote a materia medica, *De Historia Stirpium* (1542) with 500 plates, and also a work on the plague.

Casimir Funk

(1884–1967) Polish–American biochemist who studied dietary deficiencies, isolated thiamine and suggested the term 'vitamine'. He also isolated the first crude extract of androsterone from human urine.

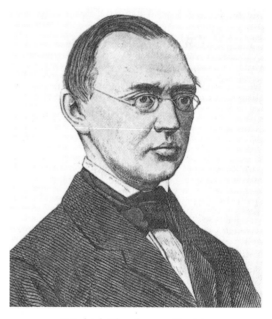

Friedrich Theodor von Frerichs

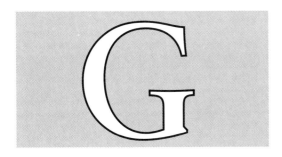

John of Gaddesden

(c 1280–1361) British physician and surgeon who wrote *Rosa Anglica Medicinae*, described windy foods, constipation and overeating at night as causes of arthritis, used a windowed bandage for inspection, and suggested light treatment for smallpox.

Georg Theodor August Gaffky

(1850–1918) German bacteriologist who was the first to isolate and culture the typhoid bacillus, discovered the cholera vibrio and studied bubonic plague in Egypt.

D Carleton Gajdusek

(b 1923) American neurologist and Nobel laureate in 1976 who worked on degenerative neurological disorders, identifying the causative agent of kuru as a 'slow virus'.

Galen

(129–200) Famous Greek doctor and prolific writer, physician to the gladiators in Rome, he studied anatomy and physiology, described osteomyelitis and scoliosis, three forms of epilepsy, muscle contraction, blood, and was the first to use the pulse as a diagnostic aid.

Galileo Galilei

(1564–1642) Italian scientist who made an early microscope and telescope, and invented a pulsilogium and a thermometer.

Franz J Gall

(1758–1828) Austrian physician and the founder of phrenology who showed that cranial nerves issue from the medulla oblongata, and considered the brain to be the source of mental activity.

WE Gallie

(1882–1959) Canadian orthopedic surgeon who developed a needle for fascial repair of hernia, and worked on cancellous grafts.

Aloysio Luigi Galvani

(1737–1798) Italian physician who discovered 'animal electricity', and wrote a book on electrical stimulation of muscles (1791).

Alfred Baring Garrod

(1819–1907) British physician who identified raised serum uric acid levels in gout patients, and introduced colchicine in the treatment of gout.

Walter Holbrook Gaskell

(1847–1914) British physiologist who identified the nerves controlling dilation of blood vessels, studied heartbeat, showed that heart muscles had intrinsic rhythmicity, and studied the sympathetic and parasympathetic nervous systems.

Herbert S Gasser

(1888–1963) American neurophysiologist who was a Nobel laureate for his work on sensory and motor nerves, and wrote *Electrical Signs of Nervous Activity* in 1937.

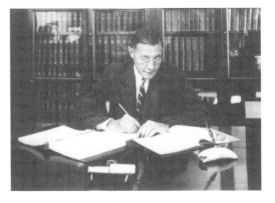

Herbert S Gasser

Karl Gegenbaur

(1826–1903) German physician and early advocate of evolutionary theory who studied comparative anatomy and the evolution of the skull.

Walter Jacob Gehring

(b 1939) Swiss geneticist who the studied genetics of *Drosophila*, and described the homeobox DNA which controls mutation and development.

William Wood Gerhard

(1809–1872) American physician who first distinguished between typhus and typhoid fevers, showing that the slow pulse and intestinal symptoms of typhoid fever were absent from typhus and contrasting the skin eruptions of the two diseases.

Walter Gilbert

(b 1932) American molecular biologist and Nobel laureate who founded the genetic engineering company, Biogen, isolated the repressor molecule controlling gene action, and described the nucleotide sequence of DNA to which it binds.

Alfred Goodman Gilman

(b 1941) American pharmacologist and Nobel laureate for his research on G proteins (named because of their activation on binding to GTP), intermediaries in pathways of cellular signalling that relay chemical messages.

Eugène Gley

(1857–1930) French endocrinologist who used oral thyroid extract, showed iodine to be present in blood and thyroid tissue, rediscovered the parathyroids and was the first to understand their significance.

Francis Glisson

(1597–1677) British physician who gave an early account of rickets and its deformities in his *De Rachitide*, produced a good anatomical description of the liver, and wrote on the 'irritability' of tissues, particularly of muscle fibers.

Themistokles Gluck

(1853–1942) German surgeon who worked on nerve suture, used synthetic tendons, and did total joint replacements using ivory and metal.

Leopold Gmelin

(1788–1853) German chemist and physiologist who studied pigmentation in the eye, and digestion. He developed Gmelin salt (potassium ferricyanide) and Gmelin test (for bile pigment), and introduced the terms 'ester' and 'ketone'.

Johann Wolfgang von Goethe

(1749–1832) German scientist and author who was the first to use the term morphology, pioneered of evolutionary theory, discovered the intermaxillary bone, and suggested that the skull was made of modified vertebrae.

Joseph Goldberger

(1874–1929) Hungarian-born American epidemiologist who studied the spread of measles, yellow fever and typhus. He investigated pellagra, showing it to be a nutritional disorder curable by addition of a protein to the diet, later shown to be niacin.

Richard Benedikt Goldschmidt

(1878–1958) German-born American molecular biologist who studied the X chromosomes and suggested (incorrectly) that they were the units of heredity. He also used heat shock to create phenocopies that mimicked genetic mutations but were not inherited.

Joseph Leonard Goldstein

(b 1940) American molecular geneticist and Nobel laureate who studied cholesterol metabolism and familial hypercholesterolemia. He found that in some diseases liver cells cannot complex with LDL because of a missing receptor site and later discovered several mutations in the LDL receptor gene.

Joel Goldthwait

(1867–1943) American orthopedic surgeon who invented a procedure for recurrent patellar displacement, and wrote on lumbar disc prolapse surgery (1911).

Camillo Golgi

(1843–1926) Italian cytologist and Nobel laureate in 1906 who developed silver nitrate staining techniques, described the intracellular Golgi apparatus, Golgi organs (nerve endings in the muscles) and worked extensively on malaria.

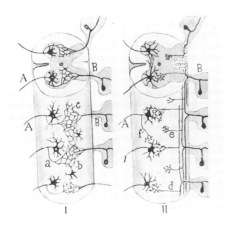

Golgi organs

Robert Gooch

(1784–1830) Outstanding British physician and midwife who wrote *An Account of Some of the Most Important Diseases peculiar to Women and Practical Midwifery*.

John Goodsir

(1814–1867) British anatomist and surgeon who applied mathematics to biology, and proposed the triangle to be the basis of natural living forms.

William Crawford Gorgas

(1854–1920) American military doctor who directed the mosquito eradication program in Havana and the Panama Canal Zone by draining swamps and covering pools with oil.

John Gorrie

(1803–1855) American physician and inventor from Florida who believed (incorrectly) that malaria and yellow fever were spread by miasms from swamps and could be controlled by cooling the air in sickrooms; he therefore invented and patented the first air conditioning unit.

Sir William R Gowers

(1845–1915) British neurologist who wrote on epilepsy in 1881, studied syphilis of the central nervous system, cerebral aneurysm, chorea, palsy, and brain injury.

Regnier de Graaf

(1641–1673) Dutch physician who wrote *On the Organs of Women..*, gave a detailed description of maturing ovarian follicles, and described the pancreas.

Albrecht von Graefe

(1828–1870) German ophthalmologist and founder of the *Archiv für Ophthalmologie*, who introduced iridectomy for glaucoma, described the von Graefe sign in thyrotoxicosis, developed the surgical correction of strabismus and cataract, described papilledema associated with intraocular tumors, and detachment of the retina.

Hans Christian Joachim Gram

(1853–1938) Danish physician who developed the Gram stain which is of fundamental importance in identifying bacteria.

Ragnar Arthur Granit

(b 1900) Finnish–Swedish neurophysiologist and Nobel laureate who studied the eye and developed the electroretinogram to study effects on retinal cells of light and color discrimination. He also researched the spinal cord and pain mechanisms.

Robert James Graves

(1796–1853) Irish physician who wrote *Clinical Lectures on the Practice of Medicine* (1848), introduced timing of the pulse with a watch, described angioneurotic edema, scleroderma, erythromelalgia, and gave a classic description of exophthalmic toxic goiter caused by hypertrophy of the thyroid – Graves disease.

Raymond Greene

(1901–1982) British endocrinologist who used radioactive iodine in goiter and also studied premenstrual syndrome.

Sir Norman McAlister Gregg

(1892–1966) Australian ophthalmologist who studied the link between German measles in pregnancy and cataracts and chorioretinopathy, as well as congenital heart disease.

Nehemiah Grew

(1641–1712) British physician who wrote *Comparative Anatomy of the Stomach and Guts and Anatomy of Plants*, he also coined the terms parenchyma and cambium, and proposed that the stamen is the male organ in the plant.

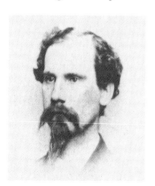

Samuel D Gross

Samuel D Gross

(1805–1884) Premier American surgeon and anatomist who introduced laparotomy for ruptured bladder, suprapubic incision for prostate disease, distinguished prostatic hypertrophy from bladder disease, and wrote *Elements of Pathological Anatomy*, which is considered the first US systematic treatise on the subject.

Ernest Hey Groves

(1872–1944) British orthopedic surgeon who wrote *Modern Methods of Treating Fractures*, detailing the use of full-thickness bone grafts.

Jules Guérin

(1801–1866) French surgeon who used tenotomy and myotomy for scoliosis and congenital hip displacement, and used plaster bandages for clubfoot.

Roger Guillemin

(b 1924) French-born American physiologist and Nobel laureate who studied the hypothalamus, isolated and identified thyrotropin-releasing hormone, growth hormone-releasing hormone and hormone-inhibiting hormone.

Sir William W Gull

(1816–1890) British endocrinologist who gave classic descriptions of myxedema, paroxysmal hemoglobinuria and anorexia nervosa.

Allvar Gullstrand

(1862–1930) Swedish ophthalmologist and Nobel prizewinner who studied physiological optics, developed mathematical formulas that are used in treatment of astigmatism and coma, and invented the slit lamp.

Irwin Clyde Gunsalus

(b 1912) American biologist who studied the metabolism of *Enterococci*, discovered pyridoxal phosphate and lipoate, used radiolabeling to elucidate the fate of carbon atoms in metabolism, and studied the cytochrome P450 system.

Sir John Bertrand Gurdon

(b 1933) British cytologist who showed that a fully differentiated cell retains the capacity and genetic information to become any other cell type, given the correct environmental stimulus.

Samuel Guthrie

(1782–1848) American chemist and physician who developed a process to convert potato starch to molasses, and distilled chloroform from chloride of lime and alcohol in a copper vessel.

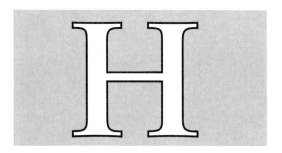

Ludwig Haberlandt

(1885–1932) Austrian endocrinologist who developed hormonal contraception and searched for a cardiac hormone.

Berthold E Hadra

(1842–1903) American orthopedic surgeon who did the first spinal fusion (1891), using silver wire to fix the spinal processes.

Waldemar Mordecai Wolff Haffkine

(1860–1930) Russian-born British microbiologist who developed a heat-killed *Vibrio cholerae* culture for protective inoculation against cholera.

Samuel Hahnemann

(1755–1843) German physician and founder of homeopathy, based on studies which showed that quinine produced malaria-type symptoms. From this he deduced that disease could be cured by drugs which cause similar symptoms to that disease.

John Scott Haldane

(1860–1936) British respiratory physiologist who developed the first respiratory gas analysis apparatus in 1898, and studied the chemical control of ventilation, stressing the importance of the partial pressure of carbon monoxide.

Stephen Hales

(1677–1761) British botanist and physiologist and the father of sphygmomanomometry who wrote *Haemastaticks*, was first to measure blood pressure,

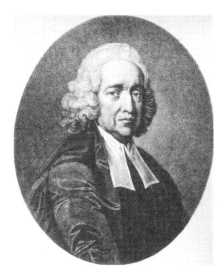

Stephen Hales

cardiac output and peripheral vascular resistance, and developed a machine for artificial ventilation.

Marshall Hall

(1790–1857) British physician and physiologist who was the first to explain the neural arc concept in reflex function and wrote on the medulla oblongata and medulla spinalis.

Albrecht von Haller

(1708–1777) German physician, early endocrinologist and neurologist who was considered the greatest physiologist of his generation. He wrote on the thyroid, precocious puberty, was the first to use the word struma, described goiter as an affection of the thymus, studied nerve and muscle action, and was the first to use the word evolution.

Edmond Halley

(1656–1742) British scientist, most remembered for the comet he discovered but also an early and important contributor to vital statistics, with his 1693 *Breslau Table of Mortality*.

William S Halsted

(1852–1922) Outstanding American surgeon who pioneered the use of antiseptics and rubber gloves in surgery, and developed techniques for breast cancer and inguinal hernia surgery.

William A Hammond

(1828–1900) American neurologist and surgeon who described athetosis, worked on snake venoms and arrow poisons, and was a founder of the US Neurological Association.

Gerhard HA Hansen

(1841–1912) Norwegian physician who devoted his life to the study of leprosy, its epidemiology, etiology, prevention and management, and discovered *Mycobacterium leprae*.

Sir Charles R Harington

(1897–1972) British endocrinologist who studied the thyroid, isolated and synthesized thyroxine, and worked on antihormones and immunochemistry.

Geoffrey W Harris

(1913–1972) British endocrinologist who studied pituitary secretions and their interaction with the brain, and showed the brain to be a target organ for ovarian hormones.

Walter Harris

(1647–1732) British pediatrician who wrote a noteworthy treatise on acute disease in infants, which included a description of the 'collection of acids' to which most childhood diseases were attributed at that time.

Ross Granville Harrison

(1870–1959) American molecular biologist who introduced the hanging-drop method of tissue culture, using it to show that nerve fibers are formed as outgrowths from nerve cells, and studied tissue grafting.

Haldan Keffer Hartline

(1903–1983) American neurologist and Nobel laureate who studied the neurophysiology of vision, analyzing the physiological stages involved in the perception of shape.

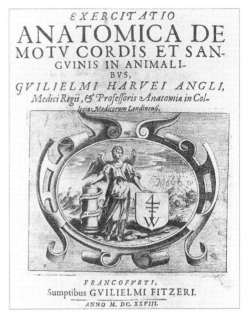

Harvey's famous treatise

William Harvey

(1578–1657) Brilliant British physician who discovered the circulation of the blood and wrote what has been described as 'the greatest treatise in the history of physiology'. He was also a pioneer in endocrinology, embryology and obstetrics.

Hakaru Hashimoto

(1881–1934) Japanese endocrinologist who described auto-immune thyroiditis with lymphocytic infiltration of the thyroid.

Clopton Havers

(c 1650–1702) British physician and anatomist who applied microscopy to the study of bone structure, and discovered the Haversian canals.

Sir Henry Head

(1861–1940) British experimental physiologist and neurologist who studied the physiology of sensation in the arm (by cutting nerves in his own arm), and wrote *Aphasia and Kindred Disorders of Speech*, based on his clinical observations of men suffering from gunshot wounds.

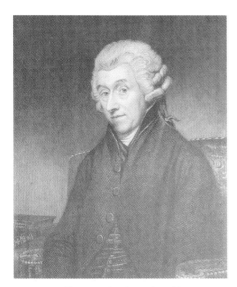

William Heberden, the elder

William Heberden, the elder

(1710–1801) Outstanding British physician who distinguished chickenpox from smallpox, described angina pectoris and finger nodules in arthritis deformans, distinguished arthritis from gout, and described nyctalopia.

William Heberden, the younger

(1767–1845) British physician who wrote *Morborum Puerilium Epitome* (1804), a classic on pediatrics, plague and fevers.

Rudolf PH Heidenhain

(1834–1897) German urologist who developed the theory of urine formation, demonstrated inorganic salts in tubular urine, and concluded that the renal tubules had a secretory function.

Jacob von Heine

(1800–1879) German neurologist and surgeon who described anterior poliomyelitis, noting its epidemic nature.

Lorenz Heister

(1683–1758) German anatomist and founder of scientific surgery who wrote an illustrated *Chirurgie*, described spinal dislocation and the thyroid as a ductless gland, did the first postmortem study of appendicitis, and introduced the term tracheotomy.

Hans Heller

(1905–1974) Czech endocrinologist who studied metabolism (particularly arginine vasotacin) and neurohypophysial hormones.

Johannes Baptiste van Helmont

(1579–1644) Flemish physician and founder of the iatrochemical school that regarded physiological and pathological phenomena as chemical in origin, coined the term gas and discovered carbon dioxide, carbon monoxide and sulfur dioxide, described lipemia in diabetes mellitus, and discovered that the stomach contains acid.

Hermann von Helmholtz

(1821–1894) German physiologist who studied the biophysics of nerves, muscle contraction, optics and color theory, and invented the ophthalmoscope.

Philip S Hench

(1896–1965) American endocrinologist and Nobel laureate who studied rheumatic fever, and was the first to use cortisone in the treatment of rheumatoid arthritis.

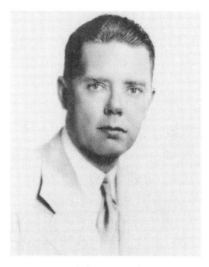

Philip S Hench

Lawrence Joseph Henderson

(1878–1942) Distinguished American physiologist and biochemist who studied acid–base equilibrium in relation to blood and body fluids and developed the Henderson–Hasselbalch equation.

Friedrich GJ Henle

(1809–1885) Greatest German histologist of his time who described the loop of the nephron, wrote on the suprarenals, the pituitary, epithelial tissues, on ovarian function and erection.

Christian Andreas Viktor Hensen

(1835–1924) German physiologist who studied hearing, and discovered Hensen ducts and Hensen supporting cells in the ear.

Herophilus

(c 335–280 BC) Greek anatomist who described the spleen, liver, brain, sex organs, nervous and vascular systems, and suggested that the brain was the center of reason and controlled the nerves, and also wrote a treatise on midwifery.

James B Herrick

(1861–1954) American physician who described the appearance of the red blood cells in sickle-cell anemia and the clinical manifestations of coronary vascular disease.

Alfred Day Hershey

(1908–1997) American microbiologist, Nobel laureate and a founder of the Phage Group, who provided conclusive proof that DNA was the genetic code material.

Walter Rudolf Hess

(1881–1973) Swiss physiologist and Nobel prizewinner who studied the mechanisms of blood pressure and heart rate regulation, particularly in relation to respiration, used microelectrodes to stimulate parts of the brain, and showed that stimulation of the hypothalamus affected respiration, sleep, blood pressure, arousal and anger.

William Hewson

(1739–1774) British surgeon and anatomist who researched the lymphatic system, described blood coagulation and properties of lymphocytes, and suggested paracentesis for correction of pneumothorax.

Corneille Jean François Heymans

(1892–1968) Belgian physiologist and Nobel laureate who showed that respiration rate is controlled by nerves, and that the aorta and carotid arteries contain cells sensitive to blood pressure and blood chemicals which are involved in the control of respiration.

Nathaniel Highmore

(1613–1685) British physician who suggested that the suprarenal glands absorbed human exudates from the large vessels, and described the maxillary sinus.

Fabricius Hildanus

(1560–1634) Brilliant German surgeon and anatomist who provided the first illustration of scoliotic spine, showed that head injury can cause insanity, invented instruments, described extraction of a foreign steel body in the eye using a magnet, and introduced the practice of amputation above the gangrenous area in a limb.

Archibald Vivian Hill

(1886–1977) Pioneer British physiologist and Nobel laureate who studied neuron and muscle activity and heat generation in relation to muscle contraction and production and use of lactic acid.

Hippocrates

(460–377 BC) Father of medicine, a Greek physician and teacher whose oath and *Aphorisms* are still relevant today, he described fractures, dislocations, painkillers, trephining, smallpox, 'sacred disease' or epilepsy, kidney disease, and many other diseases and procedures.

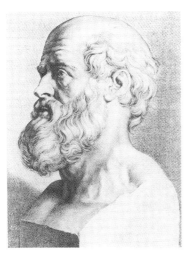

Hippocrates

Wilhelm His, Sr

(1831–1904) Swiss anatomist who studied histogenesis of the lymphatic and nervous systems, developed the microtome and use of photography, and provided the first accurate description of the human embryo.

Wilhelm His, Jr

(1863–1934) Swiss physician and anatomist who described the bundle of His, specialized fibers in the heart involved in electrical conduction from the atrioventricular node to the ventricles.

George Herbert Hitchings

(b 1905) American biochemist and Nobel laureate who developed the folic acid antagonist, 2-amino-purine, followed by allopurinol and several anti-cancer drugs, including the ant-leukemia drug, 6-mercaptopurine and the immunosuppressive drug, azathioprine. His laboratory also produced acyclovir and the anti-AIDS drug zidovudine.

Julius Eduard Hitzig

(1838–1907) German neurologist and psychiatrist who used cerebral electrophysiology and ablation techniques, finding specific areas for motor control, and studied the visual cortex.

Mahlon Bush Hoagland

(b 1921) American biochemist who studied causes of cancer, liver regeneration and growth control, provided confirmation of Crick's adaptor hypothesis of protein synthesis and discovered transfer RNA.

Nathaniel Hodges

(1629–1688) British physician who tended plague victims in London and described the clinical symptoms, treatment and means of prevention in his *Loimologia*.

Sir Alan L Hodgkin

(b 1914) British physiologist and Nobel laureate in 1963 for work on the chemistry and mathematics of nerve impulse conduction, and also described action potentials produced during cell discharge.

Thomas Hodgkin

(1798–1866) British physician who described the glandular 'Hodgkin disease' with enlargement of spleen, liver and lymphatic glands. He also described aortic insufficiency (1829), and introduced the stethoscope into the UK.

Joseph Hodgson

(1788–1869) British cardiologist who wrote a treatise on the *Diseases of Arteries and Veins* in 1815, and described cylindrical dilatation of the aorta without saccular aneurysmal bulging.

Friedrich Hoffmann

(1660–1742) German physician who described chlorosis in 1730, and rubella in 1740.

Robert William Holley

(1922–1993) American biochemist, Nobel laureate and member of the team which synthesized penicillin, he studied leucyl transfer RNAs and found two with different codons thus providing evidence of degeneracy of the amino acid code.

Sir Gordon M Holmes

(1876–1965) Leading British neurologist who wrote

Spinal Injuries of Warfare, and *Examination of the Nervous System*, and did outstanding work on the physiology of the visual cortex, the thalamus, and the cerebellum.

Oliver Wendell Holmes

(1809–1894) American physician and writer who introduced regular use of the stethoscope and achromatic microscope into teaching and practice, studied puerperal fever and recommended hygiene precautions in hospitals for its prevention.

Francis Home

(1719–1813) British physician and experimentalist who developed the first measles vaccine, described the composition of diabetic urine and the appearance of coagulated blood in fever patients.

Robert Hooke

(1635–1703) Brilliant British experimental philosopher who developed the early compound microscope, wrote *Micrographia*, described cells as biological units, used artificial respiration and blood transfusion in a dog, and designed a hearing aid.

James Hope

(1801–1841) British cardiologist and early advocate of auscultation who advanced knowledge of heart murmurs, aneurysm and valvular disease, and wrote *Diseases of the Heart and Great Vessels* (1831).

Sir Frederick G Hopkins

(1861–1947) British biochemist who wrote *On the Estimation of Uric Acid in Urine*, studied protein hydrolysis, isolated tryptophan, showed that lactic acid was a product of muscle contraction, and was a Nobel laureate in 1929 for work on the need for vitamins in normal growth.

Lemuel Hopkins

(1750–1801) Eminent American physician who was an authority on the treatment of tuberculosis, recommending fresh air and exercise, and was also a noted political satirist.

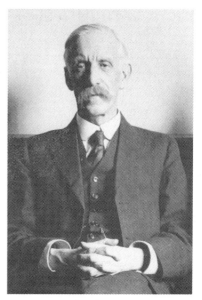

Sir Frederick G Hopkins

Felix Hoppe-Seyler

(1825–1895) German biochemist who discovered hemoglobin and named it, showed that it bound oxygen, and determined the absorption spectrum of blood containing carbon monoxide.

William E Horner

(1793–1853) American surgeon and anatomist who wrote the first US treatise on pathological anatomy, described the tensor tarsi muscle in the lachrymal apparatus, and the small muscle in the internal commisure of the eyelid, which are named after him.

Sir Victor Horsley

(1857–1916) British surgeon and physiologist who used intracranial surgery in the treatment of epilepsy, studied the effect of anesthetics on the brain, thyroid function, and rabies treatment.

David Hosack

(1769–1835) Exemplary American physician and teacher who was one of the first in the US to treat hydrocele by injection and to use ligation for a femoral artery aneurysm.

Sir Godfrey Newbold Hounsfield

(b 1919) British electrical engineer and Nobel laureate who helped to develop computer-assisted tomography (CAT) which provides detailed X-ray pictures of soft tissues of the body.

Bernardo A Houssay

(1887–1971) Argentinian physiologist and Nobel laureate who studied pituitary extracts, carbohydrate metabolism, arrhythmias, diabetes, and neurophysiology.

John Howard

(1726–1790) British reformer of conditions in prisons and hospitals (relating death rate to degree of crowding), and was responsible for instigating measures to control jail fever.

Wang Hsi

(c 1475) Chinese physician who wrote I Lin Chi Yao, describing thyroid gland position in body, and used animal gland as treatment.

David Hunter Hubel

(b 1926) Canadian neurophysiologist and Nobel laureate who studied visual perception by implanting electrodes in the brain, and analyzing individual cell responses to different visual stimuli.

Charles Brenton Huggins

(b 1901) Canadian surgeon who studied hormone treatment of cancers, particularly of the prostate and the breast, and was a Nobel laureate in 1966.

John Hughes

(b 1942) British pharmacological biochemist who discovered enkephalins, natural opiates occurring in the brain, and studied the biochemistry and pharmacology of many neuroactive compounds.

John Hunter

(1728–1793) Outstanding British surgeon, considered the founder of scientific surgery, who suggested the plastic nature of bone and noted the

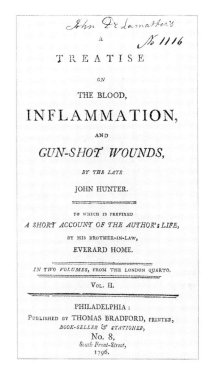

Hunter's treatise on gun-shot wounds

influence of muscle action on the skeleton, he investigated venereology, embryology, dentistry and aneurysms, amassing a huge number of pathological specimens, the basis of his famous museum.

William Hunter

(1718–1783) Eminent British anatomist and obstetrician who wrote *Anatomy of the Human Gravid Uterus*, in 1774, and described separate maternal and fetal circulations.

George Sumner Huntington

(1850–1916) American physician who was the first to recognise the hereditary chronic adult chorea named after him.

Sir Arthur Hurst

(1879–1944) British gastroenterologist who used X-rays to study movements in the stomach, intestine and colon, and studied duodenal ulcers, achalasia and constipation.

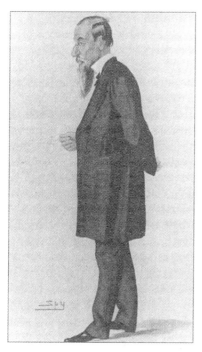

Sir Jonathan Hutchinson

several types of lupus. He also described temporal arteritis and gouty arthritis, and the eponymous triad of congenital syphilis (interstitial keratitis, notched teeth and deafness).

Ulrich von Hutten

(1488–1523) German humanist and epidemiologist who studied syphilis, describing it in The French Disease and reported the use of mercury and guaiac for it.

John Huxham

(1692–1768) British physician who wrote *An Essay on Fevers and their various kinds* (1755) giving descriptions of typhus and typhoid and the use of cinchona tincture. He also made observations on the soft palate in diphtheria, and Devonshire colic.

Sir Andrew F Huxley

(b 1917) British physiologist and Nobel laureate for work on nerve conduction and the physiology of muscle fibers, postulating a 'sliding filament' theory of muscle contraction.

Sir Jonathan Hutchinson

(1828–1913) Prolific British surgeon who made observations in many areas including ophthalmology and dermatology, he published an Atlas of Skin Diseases in which he described sarcoidosis and

Joseph Hyrtl

(1810–1894) Austrian anatomist who studied in detail the anatomy of the ear and wrote *Handbook of Topographical Anatomy*, one of the first in the German language.

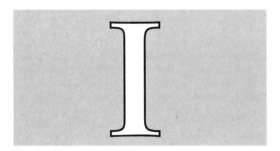

Giovanni Filippo Ingrassias

(1510–1580) Italian physician who gave the first description of the stapes and also described scarlet fever and varicella.

Alick Isaacs

(1921–1967) British microbiologist who discovered interferon in his research on the effects of interaction between influenza viruses.

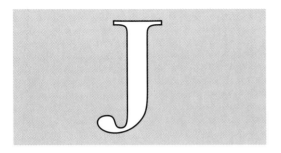

John Hughlings Jackson

(1835–1911) British neurologist and the father of modern neurology who wrote on epilepsy, stroke, and speech defects, and on the concept of 'levels' in the nervous system.

François Jacob

(b 1920) French geneticist and Nobel laureate who discovered that genes are turned on and off by other genes thus regulating each other, and formulated the operon system of repressor and operator actions.

Henry L Jaffe

(1896–1979) American pathologist, who studied bones and the endocrine system, and wrote on bone tumors and metabolic and inflammatory diseases.

Sir Alec John Jeffreys

(b 1950) British molecular biologist who developed DNA fingerprinting using restriction endonucleases and gel electrophoresis, a technique now widely used in forensic work.

Edward Jenner

(1749–1823) British physician who was responsible for the introduction of preventative inoculation – for smallpox, and also first described an anaphylactic reaction to vaccine.

Niels Kai Jerne

(1911–1994) British–Danish immunologist and Nobel laureate who examined antibody specificity and development of T-lymphocytes. He also formulated the network theory of interacting lymphocytes and antibodies.

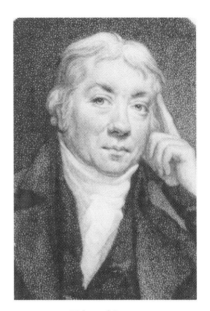

Edward Jenner

John Jones

(1729–1791) American surgeon, obstetrician and lithotomist who held the first chair of surgery and wrote the first surgical textbook in the American colonies, *Plain . . . Remarks on the Treatment of Wounds and Fractures*, in 1775.

Robert Jones

(1857–1933) British orthopedic surgeon and founder of orthopedic hospitals, who advocated the immediate reduction of fractures which dramatically reduced war deaths.

Johann CG Jörg

(1779–1856) German surgeon and obstetrician who wrote the first orthopedics textbook, and distinguished the curvature of scoliosis from spinal TB.

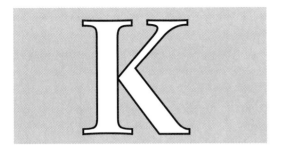

Martin David Kamen

(b 1913) Canadian-born American biochemist who pioneered the isolation and use of radioisotopes, using them in studies of photosynthesis, nitrogen fixation, calcium exchange in squamous cell carcinoma, and studies of bacterial ferridoxins.

Moritz Kaposi

(1837–1902) Leading Hungarian dermatologist who described many skin diseases including diabetic dermatitis, impetigo herpetiformis, rhinoscleroma, and malignant, multifocal reticulosis (Kaposi sarcoma).

Sir Bernard Katz

(b 1911) German-born British neurophysiologist and Nobel laureate in 1970 for work on acetylcholine, he discovered the role of calcium ions in neuro-transmission.

William W Keen

(1837–1932) American neurologist and surgeon who did the first successful removal of a brain tumor in 1888.

Edward Calvin Kendall

(1886–1972) American biochemist and Nobel laureate who isolated thyroxine and described its properties, he also isolated cortisone and related steroids.

Sir John Cowdery Kendrew

(1917–1997) British molecular biologist and Nobel laureate who used X-ray crystallography to determine the structure of myoglobin.

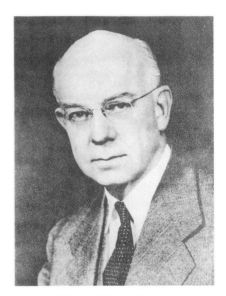

Edward Calvin Kendall

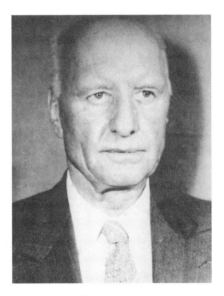

Robert F Kennedy

Robert F Kennedy

(1884–1952) American neurologist who was the first to describe shellshock as a form of hysteria, the Foster Kennedy syndrome of unilateral optic atrophy and contralateral papilledema with or without anosmia in frontal lobe tumor, and studied tumors of the hypothalamus.

Johannes Kepler

(1571–1630) German scientist and astronomer who wrote *Ad Vitellionem Paralipomena*, which included a treatise on vision, the role of the retina in sight, the lens in refraction, and myopia.

Har Gobind Khorana

(b 1922) Indian-born American molecular chemist and Nobel laureate who determined nucleic acid sequences for the 20 amino acids of the human body and their stop and start codons, and was the first to synthesize a gene artificially.

Thomas W King

(1809–1847) British physician and the father of endocrinology who described thyroid follicles and colloid of the thyroid, showing that it passed through the lymphatics and entered the great veins.

Athanasius Kircher

(1601–1680) German Jesuit scholar who was the first to use the microscope in investigating causes of disease, wrote *Scrutinium Pestis*, and described 'worms' in the blood in plague.

Baron Shibasaburo Kitasato

(1852–1931) Japanese bacteriologist who isolated the first pure culture of tetanus bacillus, discovered antitoxic immunity and also discovered the bacilli of bubonic plague, symptomatic anthrax and dysentery.

Edwin Klebs

(1834–1913) Important German pathologist and bacteriologist who developed media and methods for bacterial identification, isolated a bacillus from the brains, lungs, liver, heart and kidneys of patients, *Corynebacterium diphtheriae*, the organism responsible for diphtheria, and later isolated the typhoid bacillus and *Treponema pallidum* of syphilis.

Sir Aaron Klug

(b 1926) Lithuanian-born British molecular biologist and Nobel laureate who elucidated the structure of several viruses, including polio.

Albert Jan Kluyver

(1888–1956) Dutch biochemist who discovered that hydrogen transfer in oxidation is necessary for all metabolic processes.

Robert Koch

(1843–1910) German pioneer bacteriologist and Nobel prizewinner who studied the anthrax bacillus and showed it to be the sole cause of the disease, discovered the tuberculosis bacillus and cholera bacillus, and developed a series of essential scientific principles known as 'Koch postulates'.

Emil Theodor Kocher

(1841–1917) Swiss surgeon and Nobel laureate who worked on the surgical treatment of thyroid disorders, including tumors and goiter, described post-operative hypothyroidism and also pioneered operations of the brain and spinal cord.

Georges Jean Franz Köhler

(1946–1995) German immunochemist and Nobel laureate who undertook the first production of hybridomas and monoclonal antibodies, and also studied immunoglobulins and their structural mutants.

Willem Johan Kolff

(b 1911) Dutch-born American physician who developed the first rotating drum artificial kidney or dialysis machine, and did research on the heart–lung machine.

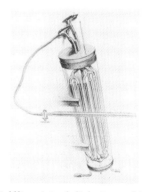

Kolff's original dialysis machine

Rudolph Albert von Kölliker

(1817–1905) Swiss anatomist and morphologist who studied cell structure and embryology, his studies established cytology as a separate specialty.

Franz König

(1832–1910) German hematologist and surgeon who identified the relationship between hemophilia and hemophilic arthropathy and described three stages in the disease.

Arthur Kornberg

(b 1918) American molecular biologist and Nobel laureate who discovered DNA polymerase, showed that DNA synthesis requires a template DNA and base pairing to produce the helical structure, and was the first to synthesize viral DNA.

Sergei S Korsakoff

(1854–1900) Russian neurologist and neuro-psychiatrist who described a syndrome of alcoholic neuropathy with loss of memory for recent events.

Albrecht Kossel

(1853–1927) German biochemist and Nobel prizewinner who isolated nuclein, protein and nucleic acid from the nucleus of spermatozoa, and also showed that nucleic acid contained the four bases of DNA, discovering adenine, thymidine, cytosine and uracil.

Edwin Gerhard Krebs

(b 1918) American biochemist and Nobel laureate who discovered phosphorylase kinase and phosphatase, elucidating the phosphorylation cascade that switches on glycogen phosphorylase and other enzymes under the influence of hormones such as glucagon and epinephrine.

Sir Hans Adolf Krebs

(1900–1981) German-born British biochemist and Nobel laureate who described the urea cycle and the citric acid cycle (Krebs cycle) of energy production, and also studied ketone bodies and purine synthesis.

August Krogh

(1874–1949) Eminent Danish physiologist and Nobel laureate who studied respiration and the capillary system showing that surrounding muscle tissue activity affects the blood flow through capillaries, and later that they were under nervous and hormonal control.

Karl Hugo Kronecker

(1839–1914) Leading German physiologist who invented the frog-heart manometer, a perfusion cannula and other instruments, advanced the all-or-none principle of cardiac muscle, and studied the transmission of esophageal contractions and the effects of altitude.

Stephen William Kuffler

(1913–1980) American neurobiologist who studied synaptic transmission, retinal physiology and the electrophysiology of glial cells.

Wilhelm Kühne

(1837–1900) German physiologist who studied digestion, proposed the term 'enzyme', showed rigor mortis to be caused by the action of myosin, and discovered rhodopsin and its photoreversibility in animal experiments.

Adolf Kussmaul

(1822–1902) German physician who did the first esophagogastroscopy, described periarteritis nodosa, paradoxical pulse, progressive bulbar palsy, and observed diabetic coma with ketosis and air-hunger (Kussmaul breathing).

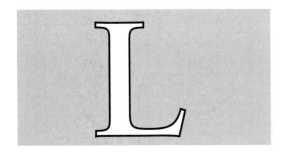

Rene TH Laennec

(1781–1826) French physician who invented the monoaural stethoscope, described heart and lung sounds and murmurs, and studied pulmonary disease.

Albin Lambotte

(1866–1955) Belgian surgeon and the first to operate for gastric ulcer, who performed early craniotomy, introduced osteosynthesis, and developed instruments for it.

Giovanni Maria Lancisi

(1654–1720) Italian physician and a great epidemiologist who described epidemics of influenza, cattle plague, and malaria suggesting that it was caused by mosquitoes, he also wrote on aneurysms, and on sudden death.

Karl Landsteiner

(1868–1943) American pathologist and Nobel laureate, founder of serology, who introduced the blood grouping system which revolutionized blood transfusion.

Sir W Arbuthnot Lane

(1856–1943) British orthopedic surgeon who wrote a pioneering book, *Operative Treatment of Fractures*, was the first to use metal plates rather than wires to join fractures and devised the 'no-touch' operative technique and an operation for cleft palate.

Paul Langerhans

(1847–1888) German physician and pathologist who described dendritic cells in skin, and the islets of the pancreas.

John Newport Langley

(1852–1925) British physiologist who studied the secretory activity of glandular tissues, the action of pilocarpine on the heart, and showed that sympathetic nerve fibers were single units and that a ganglion was a relay station.

Dominique-Jean Larrey

(1766–1842) Famous French orthopedic and military surgeon who wrote on gunshot wounds, formed a 'flying' ambulance service, studied spinal caries, and was the first to amputate through the hip joint.

Charles Louis Alphonse Laveran

(1845–1922) French physician and Nobel laureate who discovered the malarial parasite, suggested transmission via mosquito bites, and also studied sleeping sickness, kala-azar and leishmaniasis.

Antoine Laurent Lavoisier

(1743–1794) French scientist who discovered oxygen, described its importance in respiration and the interchange of gases in the lungs, likened respiration to combustion, and developed quantitative chemistry.

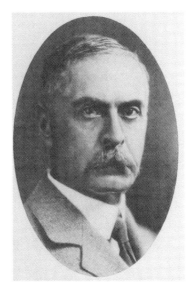

Karl Landsteiner

Thomas Laycock

(1812–1876) British anatomist and proponent of public health and vital statistics who formulated a theory that the entire nervous system functions on a reflex pattern and wrote his major work, *Mind and Brain*, in 1859.

Philip Leder

(b 1934) American geneticist who discovered the arrangement, and coding and non-coding regions, of globin genes on the chromosome, studied the function of oncogenes and developed and patented the 'oncomouse'.

Joshua Lederberg

(b 1925) American geneticist and Nobel laureate who discovered conjunction and transduction in bacteria, introduced replica plating, and made important discoveries about the breeding of viruses and their effect on bacteria.

Antoni van Leeuwenhoek

(1632–1723) Dutch microscopist and father of protozoology and bacteriology, he built over 200 simple microscopes, described protozoa, bacteria, blood corpuscles, and spermatozoa, and the striated fibers found in bundles in voluntary muscles.

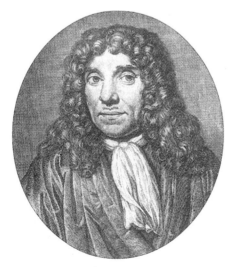

Antoni van Leeuwenhoek

Sir William Boog Leishman

(1865–1926) British physician who discovered the protozoan parasite of kala-azar and developed a stain for its detection, he also developed a vaccine against typhoid.

Luis Frederico Leloir

(1906–1987) French-born Argentinian biochemist and Nobel laureate who discovered angiotensin and studied glucose metabolism and glycogen storage.

François Jules Lemaire

(1814–1886) French biochemist who described the antiseptic properties of phenol.

Nicolas Lémery

(1645–1715) French chemist and pharmacist who wrote an influential book *Cours de chymie* containing details of methods and classification of compounds.

Nicolo Leonicenus

(1428–1524) Italian physician who wrote one of the earliest treatises on syphilis, described syphilitic hemiplegia and blindness, and corrected botanical errors in Pliny's *Natural History*.

René Leriche

(1879–1955) French surgeon who worked on surgery of the vascular system and peripheral nerve injuries, introduced periarterial sympathectomy and described a symptom complex associated with gradual occlusion of the bifurcation of the aorta.

John Coakley Lettsom

(1744–1815) British physician who described addiction to drugs and alcohol in 1786, founded the Aldgate Dispensary, and recommended artificial respiration for victims of drowning.

Phoebus Aaron Theodor Levene

(1869–1940) Russian-born American biochemist who studied nucleic acids and the ribose and deoxyribose sugars in them, described optical isomerism of organic substances and worked on phospholipids.

Rita Levi-Montalcini

(b 1901) Italian–American neurophysiologist and Nobel Laureate in 1986, who studied in vitro nerve growth, and discovered nerve growth factor, opening up further studies into neurological disease, tissue regeneration and cancer mechanisms.

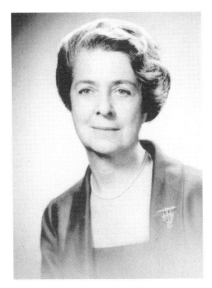

Rita Levi-Montalcini

Sir Thomas Lewis

(1881–1945) British cardiologist and clinical scientist responsible for the early use of electrocardiography, founder of the journal Heart, he wrote *Clinical Electrocardiography* in 1913.

Edward B Lewis

(b 1918) American developmental geneticist and Nobel laureate who discovered the control mechanisms in early embryonic development, showing that genes are arranged on a chromosome in the same order as in corresponding body segments.

Richard Charles Lewontin

(b 1929) American geneticist who studied variation in population genetics, developed the multi-locus theory, and introduced gel electrophoresis for protein sequencing in 1966.

Erich Lexer

(1867–1937) German orthopedic surgeon who pioneered transplantation, and maintenance of viability of tissues, including bone ends and whole joints.

Choh Hao Li

(b 1913) Chinese-born American biochemist who worked on pituitary hormones, isolated luteinizing hormone, adrenocorticotrophic hormone, somatotropin and follicle stimulating hormone.

Andreas Libavius

(c 1560–1616) German physician and chemist whose *Alchemia* was the first systematic treatise on science, he analysed mineral waters, discovered stannic chloride, and was one of the founders of the iatrochemical school.

Grant W Liddle

(1921–1989) American endocrinologist who studied the adrenals and aldosterone, regulation of ACTH and MSH secretion, hormonal control, and corticosteroid therapy.

Justus von Liebig

(1803–1873) German chemist who discovered chloroform, hippuric acid, chloral and tyrosine, studied nutrition and degradation of proteins and showed that fats and carbohydrates were oxidized in the tissues.

Clarence Walton Lillehei

(b 1918) American cardiovascular and thoracic surgeon who pioneered open-heart surgery.

Thomas Linacre

(c 1460–1524) British physician, the founder, in 1518, of the College of Physicians in London which licenced all physicians, physician to Henry VIII, translator of Leoniceno, Galen and others, he also studied muscles and locomotion.

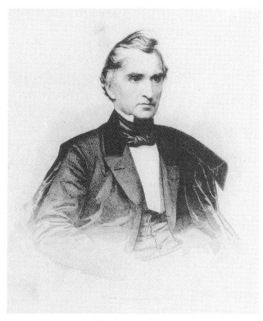

Justus von Liebig

James Lind

(1716–1794) Pioneer British naval surgeon who wrote on scurvy and its treatment with antiscorbutics such as green vegetables, wine and lemon juice, he also wrote on naval hygiene and prevention of contagious diseases, tropical medicine and malaria, for which he recommended cinchona.

Carl Linnaeus

(1707–1778) Swedish naturalist and physician and father of systematic binomial taxonomy, who wrote Systema Naturae (1735), a materia medica, a nosology, described embolism, aphasia, and the waterborne nature of malaria.

Fritz Albert Lipmann

(1899–1986) German-born American biochemist and Nobel laureate who studied phosphorylation in respiration, electron transport, discovered coenzyme A and partially elucidated its molecular structure.

Hans Lippershey

(c 1570–1619) Dutch spectacle maker who combined long and short focus convex lenses to produce a telescope, and showed that the combination when reversed becomes a microscope.

Li Shih-Chen

(1518–1593) Chinese physician and the father of Chinese herbal medicine who compiled the *Pen Tshao Kang Mu*, an early pharmacopoeia.

Lord Joseph Lister

(1827–1912) British surgeon and father of antiseptic surgery who used carbolic acid and drastically reduced death from post-operative infection.

Robert Liston

(1794–1847) British surgeon who developed a lateral splint for femoral fractures that was used for 100 years, and performed the first major operation in London under ether anesthesia.

William John Little

(1810–1894) British orthopedic surgeon who wrote *Treatise on Deformities*, and described spastic diplegia, club foot, treatment of ankylosis, and knee surgery.

Sir Charles Locock

(1799–1875) British physician and obstetrician who suggested that crowded teeth, onanism and menstruation were causes of epilepsy, and treated the disease with potassium bromide.

Otto Loewi

(1873–1961) German pharmacologist and a Nobel laureate who studied protein and carbohydrate metabolism, the autonomic nervous system, heart, kidney and pancreatic function. His major work was on the chemical transmission of nerve impulses and he discovered acetylcholine.

Friedrich August Johann Löffler

(1852–1915) German microbiologist who cultured the diphtheria bacillus, discovered the causative organisms of glanders and swine erysipelas, developed a vaccine against foot-and-mouth disease, and produced the first evidence of the existence of filterable viruses.

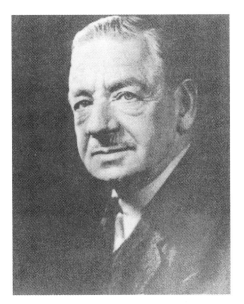

Otto Loewi

Crawford Williamson Long

(1815–1878) American physician and the first to use sulfuric ether for surgical anesthesia.

Rafael Lorente de No

(b 1902) Spanish–American neurophysiologist who studied synaptic transmission, the anatomy of neuron networks and coordination of eye movement.

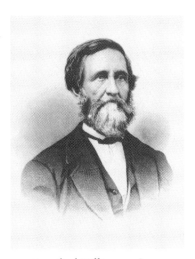

Crawford Williamson Long

Adolf Lorenz

(1854–1946) Austrian orthopedic surgeon who wrote on scoliosis, and used manipulation for congenital hip displacement.

Antoine C Lorry

(1725–1783) French physician who experimented on suboccipital and spinal puncture in animals, and showed that the medulla is the center of respiration.

Pierre CA Louis

(1787–1872) French physician and the founder of medical statistics, who worked on tuberculosis, typhoid fever (and named it), showed that bloodletting was of little value in pneumonia, and described the angle of Louis (angulus sterni).

Peter Lowe

(1550–1610) British surgeon and the founder of the Royal Faculty of Physicians and Surgeons of Glasgow who prepared the first comprehensive book on surgery in English, *The Discourse of the whole Art of Chyrurgerie*.

Richard Lower

(1631–1691) British physician and anatomist who wrote *Tractatus de Corde* on the form and function of the heart in 1669, he also wrote on the origin of catarrh, described pituitary secretions, and gave the first blood transfusion from a donor artery to a recipient's jugular vein.

Keith Lucas

(1879–1916) British neurophysiologist who studied the properties of nerves and muscles and the propagation of nerve impulses, demonstrating that a phase of reduced excitability follows the nerve impulse.

Carl FW Ludwig

(1816–1895) Pioneer German physiologist who proposed endosmosis in the glomerular membrane and studied capillary blood pressure, and the nervous system. He also devised the kymograph to study respiration and circulation, a blood gas analyzer, and a device to measure blood flow.

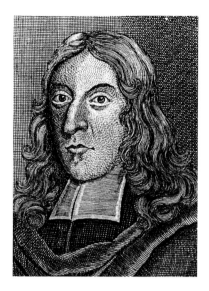

Richard Lower

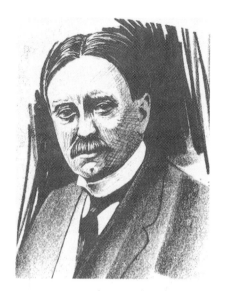

Graham Lusk

Salvador Edward Luria

(1912–1991) Italian–American microbiologist and Nobel laureate who studied the role of DNA in bacterial and phage mutations, and co-founded the Phage Group.

Graham Lusk

(1866–1932) Founder of the science of nutrition in America, who studied the influence of carbohydrates on protein metabolism in diabetes mellitus and developed a respiration calorimeter for his studies of phlorizin diabetes.

André Michel Lwoff

(b 1902) French microbiologist and Nobel laureate who studied bacterial and phage genetics, genetic control of enzymes and viral synthesis, he showed how phage DNA was incorporated into the bacterial chromosome, subsequently dividing with it (lysogeny).

Feodor Felix Konrad Lynen

(1911–1979) German biochemist and Nobel laureate who isolated coenzyme A and demonstrated its formation into acetyl-S-CoA through a thioester bond, he also studied fatty acid metabolism and cholesterol biosynthesis.

Mary Frances Lyon

(b 1925) British scientist who studied genetics and metagenesis, and a world authority on oncomouse genetics and their value in studying human hereditary diseases. Known particularly for her hypothesis that one of the two X chromosomes in female mammals is (randomly) inactivated in early development.

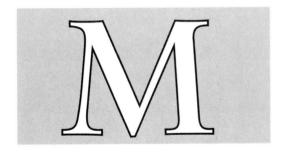

Sir William Macewen

(1848–1924) British surgeon who was one of first to operate successfully on brain tumors, abscesses and trauma, and also on spinal tumor in 1885, he pioneered bone grafting, and wrote *The Growth of Bone: Observations on Osteogenesis*.

Sir Colin MacKenzie

(1877–1938) Australian orthopedic surgeon who developed treatment of polio with muscle rest, and set up a department of muscle retraining.

Sir James Mackenzie

(1853–1925) Outstanding British cardiologist who wrote *The Study of the Pulse* which distinguished benign from critical irregularities of the heart, followed by *Diseases of the Heart*, and described the diagnosis and treatment of auricular fibrillation.

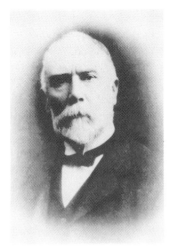

Sir James Mackenzie

Sir Morell Mackenzie

(1837–1892) Leading British laryngologist who wrote a two-volume *Manual of Diseases of the Throat and Nose*, he developed instruments and techniques including a laryngeal mirror and a laryngeal guillotine.

Jay MacLean

(1890–1957) American biochemist who isolated heparin while still a student.

John James Rickard MacLeod

(1876–1935) British physiologist and Nobel laureate who studied and wrote on carbohydrate metabolism and respiration but is best remembered for the discovery of insulin.

Dame Jean Macnamara

(1899–1968) Australian physician who worked on infantile paralysis and the polio virus, finding that there were several strains, so contributing to the development of the Salk vaccine.

François Magendie

(1783–1855) French physiologist and experimental pharmacologist who discovered alkaloid compounds, studied strychnine poisoning and emetine, anaphylaxis, and wrote *Experiments on the Function of the Roots of Spinal Nerves* in 1822.

Horace Winchell Magoun

(1907–1991) American pioneer neuroendocrinologist who studied the structure and function of the hypothalamus, and wrote *The Waking Brain* in 1963 which described his findings on brain–endocrine interactions.

Moses Maimonides

(1135–1204) Jewish–Arab physician and philosopher who wrote *Tractatus Regimine Sanitatis*, discussed dietetics and poisons, the use of drugs and gymnastics, and described amputation and asthma.

Joseph F Malgaigne

(1806–1865) French surgeon and the first in France

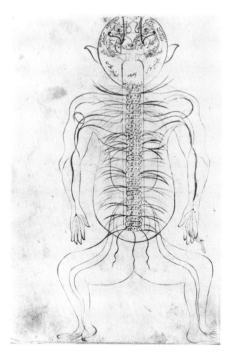

Moses Maimonides – C16 Nervous System

to use general anesthesia, he wrote on fractures, and designed the racquet incision for amputation.

Marcello Malpighi

(1628–1694) Italian physician, microscopist and founder of histology who described the embryology of a chick, graafian follicles, capillary circulation and vesicular structure of the lungs, the glomerular tufts of the kidneys and the Malphigian bodies of the spleen.

Sir Patrick Manson

(1844–1922) British physician, known as 'Mosquito Manson', who studied malaria, and the mosquito transmission of elephantiasis, wrote *Tropical Diseases* and helped to found the London School of Tropical Medicine in 1899.

Al-Mansur

(c 970) Arab physician who wrote on pharmacology, and founded a hospital in Cairo which included gynecology wards.

Pierre Marie

(1853–1940) French neurologist who described acromegaly and associated it with pituitary tumor, peroneal muscular atrophy, hypertrophic pulmonary osteoarthropathy, and cleidocranial dystostosis.

Guy F Marrian

(1904–1981) British biochemist who, in 1929, isolated estriol from human pregnant urine, studied steroid biochemistry and the sex hormones.

Edmé Marriotte

(1620–1684) French physicist who discovered the blind spot and described the function of various parts of the eye.

Francis HA Marshall

(1878–1949) British physiologist and a pioneer in reproductive physiology, he made extensive studies of the estrous cycle.

Archer John Porter Martin

(b 1910) British biochemist and Nobel laureate who worked on vitamin deficiencies and developed partition chromatography and later, gas–liquid chromatography.

George Martine

(1702–1741) British physician who wrote *Essays and Observations on the Construction and Graduation of the Thermometer*, and gave the first scientific treatise on the importance of body temperature.

Antonius Mathysen

(1805–1878) Dutch orthopedic surgeon who invented the plaster of Paris bandage.

François Mauriceau

(1637–1709) French obstetrician who wrote an illustrated book on diseases of pregnant and puerperal women (1668) which gives descriptions of normal labor, the use of version, and placenta previa. He was the first to describe tubal pregnancy and epidemic puerperal fever.

Leo Mayer

(1884–1972) American orthopedic surgeon and pioneer in reconstructive tendon operations for polio, he also studied bone tumors.

Sir Theodore Turquet de Mayerne

(1573–1655) Franco-British physician who used chemical agents in treatment, including calomel and mercurial ointments, he wrote 23 volumes including works on arthritis, obstetrics and pharmacy.

John Mayow

(1643–1679) British physiologist and chemist who demonstrated that dark venous blood is changed to bright red blood by taking something from the air, calling it nitroaerian particles, he also studied the function of intercostal muscles and the spine, fetal nutrition and rickets.

Earl D McBride

(1891–1975) American orthopedic surgeon who developed hallux valgus surgery, and a system for rating disability.

Charles McBurney

(1845–1913) American surgeon and gastrologist who studied appendicitis and showed sepsis only

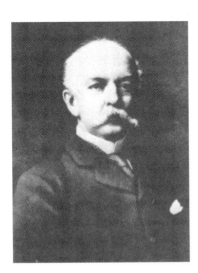

Charles McBurney

occurred following perforation, and named the point of maximum tenderness in acute appendicitis.

George McClellan

(1796–1847) Leading American surgeon and anatomist who developed procedures for ligation of the innominate artery, dissection of the clavicle, and extirpation of the parotid gland.

Barbara McClintock

(1902–1992) American scientist and Nobel laureate who produced the ultimate proof of the chromosome theory of heredity, and discovered the 'transposon' or controlling element of genes.

Elmer Verner McCollum

(1879–1967) American biochemist who gave the first description of an accessory food factor – vitamin, distinguishing between fat-soluble (A) and water-soluble (B) vitamins. He discovered vitamin D which prevents rickets, vitamin A1, A2, and nicotinamide.

Ephraim McDowell

(1771–1830) American surgeon, frontier physician and the first to successfully remove an ovarian cyst (weighing more than 20 pounds!).

Dame Anne Laura McLaren

(b 1927) British geneticist who worked on embryology, immunology and reproduction, and discovered and isolated the embryonal carcinoma cell line now used to study the differentiation of cells and the nature of cancer growth.

Richard Mead

(1673–1754) British physician who wrote on poisons and on the scabies mite as a pathological agent, advocated quarantine, and inoculated the Royal family against smallpox.

Johann F Meckel, the elder

(1724–1774) German physician who discovered the Meckel ganglion of the 5th cranial nerve, gave the first description of the submandibular ganglion, and studied the nerve supply to the face.

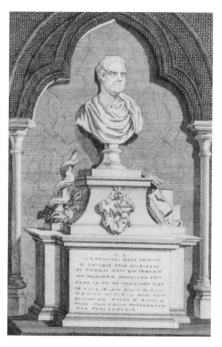

Memorial to Richard Mead

Johann F Meckel, the younger

(1781–1833) German surgeon and greatest anatomist of the period, who studied human abnormalities, wrote a comparative anatomy and other books, and described Meckel diverticulum of the intestine.

Philipp T Meckel

(1756–1803) German physician and obstetrician who studied the internal ear, and edited the Archiv der practischen *Arzenkunst*.

Sir Peter Brian Medawar

(1915–1987) British immunologist and Nobel laureate who studied skin grafting and transplant rejection and showed that the immunological response was similar to the reaction to foreign bodies.

Job van Meekeren

(1611–1666) Dutch physician and orthopedic surgeon who gave the first description of torticollis.

Joseph Vincent Meigs

(1892–1963) American gynecologist who described an eponymous syndrome of ovarian tumor associated with ascites and pleural effusion.

Georg Meissner

(1829–1905) German histologist whose name is associated with two eponyms: the submucosal plexus of the intestine and a sensory end-organ in skin (Meissner corpuscles). He also studied mesenteric plexus regulation of glandular secretions.

Sir Edward Mellanby

(1884–1955) British pharmacologist who studied nutrition and the role of vitamins, advocated cod-liver oil (vitamin D) for rickets, and showed that vitamin A deficiency caused embryonic nerve and bone malformations.

Lady May Mellanby

(1882–1978) British scientific nutritionalist who studied dental development and showed the importance of vitamins A and D in tooth formation.

Johann Gregor Mendel

(1822–1884) Pioneer Austrian botanist and geneticist who discovered the mechanism of inheritance, and is considered the founder of genetics.

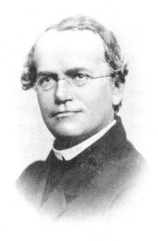

Johann Gregor Mendel

Chi-Mao Meng

(1897–1980) Chinese orthopedic surgeon who devised an abduction osteotomy of the upper femur for treatment of old unreduced congenital hip displacement in adults.

Prosper Menière

(1799–1862) French physician and otolaryngologist who showed that vertigo, nausea, tinnitus and unilateral deafness were caused by a lesion in the labyrinth of the ear.

Hieronymous Mercurialis

(1530–1606) Italian physician who produced the first illustrated book on sports medicine, the first systematic treatise on dermatology, one on pediatrics and another on ear disease.

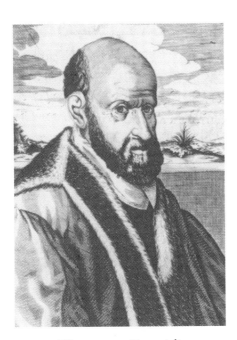

Hieronymous Mercurialis

Matthew Stanley Meselson

(b 1930) American molecular biologist who studied DNA replication (and showed it to be conservative), DNA repair and methylation, recombination, and the effects of heat shock.

Franz Anton Mesmer

(1734–1815) Austrian physician who, while experimenting with a magnet, thought that similar powers could be found in the human mind – so developed mesmerism, the forerunner of hypnotism.

Elie Metchnikoff

(1845–1916) Russian microbiologist and Nobel laureate who discovered phagocytosis, suggested the role of macrophages in attacking invading bacteria, and later investigated aging and death.

Otto Fritz Meyerhof

(1884–1951) American biochemist and Nobel laureate who studied the bioenergetics and metabolic pathways of muscle contraction, and elucidated the Embden–Meyerhof pathway of glycolysis.

Johann von Mikulicz-Radecki

(1850–1905) Polish surgeon who developed the gastroscope and esophagoscope, was the first to suture perforated gastric ulcer, and introduced the use of the gauze mask for surgeons, and described a syndrome of enlargement of lacrymal and salivary glands.

Jacques FAP Miller

(b 1931) French-born Australian immunologist who worked on the thymus and showed it to be important in the control of the immune response, and the site of T lymphocyte cell production.

Cesar Milstein

(b 1927) Argentinian–British molecular biologist and Nobel laureate who worked on the production of antibodies and developed hybridomas, from which he produced monoclonal antibodies.

Oskar Minkowski

(1858–1931) Russian–German pathologist who studied purine metabolism, acromegaly, diabetic coma, and discovered (with von Mehring) that pancreatectomy causes diabetes mellitus.

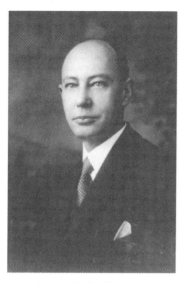

George Richards Minot

George Richards Minot

(1885–1950) American hematologist and Nobel laureate who developed staining techniques for diagnosis of anemias and a raw liver diet in pernicious anemia, and identified the role of bone marrow in red cell production.

Silas Weir Mitchell

(1829–1914) American neurologist who wrote on headache and its relationship to astigmatism and erythromelagia, and treated hysteria and nervous exhaustion.

Constantin von Monakow

(1853–1930) Russian neurologist who investigated higher centers of the nervous system, and the extra-pyramidal nervous system, and confirmed the origin of the optic nerve in the retina, and discovered the cunneate nucleus and the rubrospinal tract.

Henri de Mondeville

(c 1260–1320) French anatomist and surgeon and a prolific writer, he described aseptic treatments, bandages and splints for fractures, wrote a materia medica, and divided diseases into those caused by accidents and those of intrinsic or unknown cause.

Mondino de Luzzi

(1275–1326) Italian anatomist and physician who wrote *Anathomia Mundini* in 1316, performed early human cadaver dissections, described the pancreas and differences between the virgin and multiparae uterus.

Jacques Lucien Monod

(1910–1976) French molecular biologist and Nobel laureate who developed the operon theory of gene control, and coined the term messenger RNA (mRNA).

Alexander Monro

(1697–1767) British surgeon and founder of a dynasty of anatomists who held the chair of anatomy in Edinburgh for 126 years, he wrote *Osteology*, and *Observations Anatomical and Physiological.*

Alexander Monro

(1733–1817) British anatomist and physician who studied the lymphatics, showing them to be an

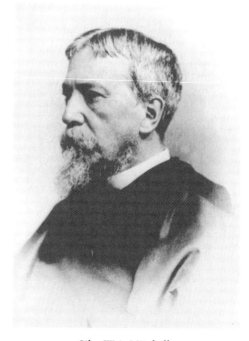

Silas Weir Mitchell

absorbent system separate from the blood circulation, he developed the paracentesis operation for pneumothorax, and wrote on the nervous system, the eye and ear. He described the foramen of Monro, a communication between the lateral ventricles and the brain.

Luc Montagnier

(b 1932) French molecular biologist who discovered and isolated the HIV virus.

Stanford Moore

(1913–1982) American biochemist and Nobel prizewinner who developed column chromatography for amino acid analysis and an automatic analyzer for RNA sequencing.

Giovanni B Morgagni

(1682–1771) Italian physician and anatomist and founder of modern morbid anatomy, he discovered the glands of the trachea, described the male urethra and female genitalia, syphilitic aneurysm and tumors, and endocranial hyperostosis, cardiac valvular lesions and tuberculosis of the kidney.

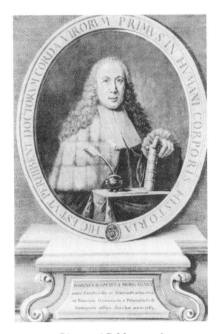

Giovanni B Morgagni

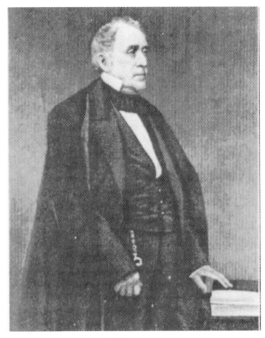

Valentine Mott

John Morgan

(1735–1789) American physician and founder of the first US medical school at the College of Philadelphia in 1765, who wrote the first treatise on improving medical education in the US.

Richard Morton

(1637–1698) British physician who wrote a comprehensive treatise on tuberculosis that described its rapid spread, symptoms of jaundice, arthritis, weight loss and intermittent fever and the recommendation of fresh air for prevention.

Valentine Mott

(1785–1865) Leading (and ambidextrous) American surgeon who used ligatures on the great vessels, did the first total excision of the clavicle, and was a founder of the New York Academy of Medicine.

Vernon Benjamin Mountcastle

(b 1918) American neurophysiologist who studied sensation and perception, his work contributed to a better understanding of memory and learning ability.

Berkeley GA Moynihan

(1865–1936) Brilliant British surgeon who studied gallstones, developed techniques in stomach, pancreas and abdominal surgery, and differentiated gastric from duodenal ulcers.

Hermann Joseph Müller

(1890–1967) American geneticist and Nobel laureate who used X-rays to induce genetic mutations, used these to verify the chromosome theory of heredity, proposed safety measures for the use of radiation in hospitals and campaigned against nuclear bomb tests.

Johannes Peter Müller

(1801–1858) German pioneering physiologist who studied embryology, phonation, and color vision, and proposed a law of specific nerve energies where the response of each sensory system will be the same whether the stimulus is chemical, thermal, mechanical or electric.

Kary Banks Mullis

(b 1944) American biochemist and Nobel laureate who discovered the polymerase chain reaction that allows the production of millions of copies of a small amount of DNA, so making analysis more practical.

John Benjamin Murphy

(1857–1916) Innovative American surgeon and teacher who developed interpositional arthroplasty for joints, but is chiefly remembered for his contribution to gastrointestinal and biliary surgery and a clinical sign of gall bladder inflammation.

William Parry Murphy

(1892–1987) American physician and Nobel prizewinner who investigated the effects of a raw liver diet in controlling pernicious anemia.

Joseph Edward Murray

(b 1919) American surgeon and Nobel laureate who did the first successful kidney transplant (between identical twins), studied immune response and methods of suppressing it using X-rays and drugs such as azathioprine.

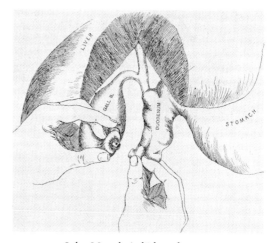

John Murphy's kidney button

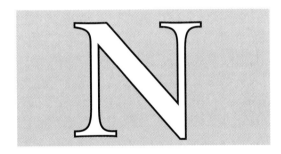

Jean Nageotte

(1866–1948) French histologist who described the boutons terminaux of spinal nerves, located the initial lesion of tabes dorsalis, and studied nerve regeneration.

Daniel Nathans

(b 1928) American geneticist and Nobel laureate who made the first genetic map, using restriction enzymes to fragment SV40 DNA, allowing identification of specific genes.

Bernhard Naunyn

(1839–1925) Gifted German endocrinologist and pathological chemist who studied metabolic diseases and the hereditary nature of diabetes mellitus.

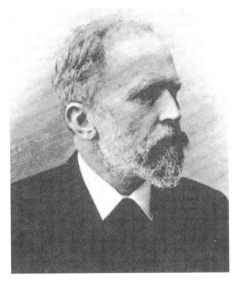

Bernhard Naunyn

Joseph Needham

(1900–1995) British biochemist who studied developmental organization in amphibians and postulated the involvement of a sterol hormone, he also wrote a history of acupuncture and a history of Chinese science.

Erwin Neher

(b 1944) German biophysicist and Nobel laureate who made the first successful recording of electric current through single ion membrane channels, and developed the patch–clamp method for biophysical measurement of small areas of a membrane which revolutionized cell physiology.

Auguste Nélaton

(1807–1873) French oncologist and surgeon who described tuberculous osteomyelitis, wrote on sarcomas and benign tumors of bone, performed ovariotomy and introduced the rubber catheter.

Charles Jules Henri Nicolle

(1866–1936) French physician, microbiologist and Nobel laureate who discovered that typhus is spread by lice, and studied the transmission, treatment and prevention of leishmaniasis, toxoplasmosis, and brucellosis.

Florence Nightingale

(1820–1910) British nurse who established a nursing service for the British army in the Crimea, developed training schools for nurses, and advocated improved hygiene conditions and the establishment of an army medical corps.

Marshall Warren Nirenberg

(b 1927) American biochemist and Nobel prizewinner who studied the 'code dictionary' of nucleotide base codons by synthesizing nucleic acid with a known base sequence and working out which amino acid it converted to protein.

Alfred Nobel

(1833–1896) Swedish chemist and industrialist who, apart from inventing dynamite and endowing the

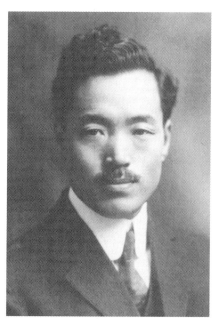

Hideyo Noguchi

Nobel Prizes, suggested the use of nitroglycerin in heart disease.

Hideyo Noguchi

(1876–1928) Japanese–American bacteriologist who was the first to culture *Treponema pallidum* which causes syphilis, then developing a skin test for it, he also found that *Bartonella bacilliformis* causes Oroya fever and is transmitted by sand flies, and proved yellow fever to be a viral disease.

Carl von Noorden

(1858–1944) German-born physician who devised a dietary regime for diabetes mellitus, and also studied the metabolism of sugar in the liver.

John Howard Northrop

(1891–1987) American biochemist and Nobel laureate who was the first to crystallize pepsin, find its molecular weight and show it to be a protein, he then purified chymotrypsin and diphtheria toxin. He isolated the first bacterial virus, and was the first to show that an enzyme's chemical properties are related to its biological activity.

Sir Gustav JV Nossal

(b 1931) Australian immunologist who studied antibody response in immunity, and discovered the one cell-one antibody rule.

Christiane Nüsslein-Volhard

(b 1942) German developmental geneticist and Nobel prizewinner for her work on the mechanisms of early embryonic development. She showed that there were three genetic categories: gap genes, pair-rule genes and segment-polarity genes.

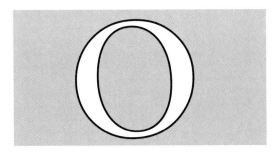

Severo Ochoa

(b 1905) American geneticist and Nobel laureate who isolated two enzymes from the Krebs cycle, studied polynucleotide phosphorylase, and elucidated the direction of protein synthesis along DNA.

Richard L O'Connor

(1933–1980) American orthopedic surgeon who did early arthroscopy of the knee, and developed instruments for meniscectomy.

Reiji Okazaki

(1930–1975) Japanese geneticist who was the first to identify the DNA–RNA fragments named after him, using these to show how DNA was synthesized simultaneously in opposing directions, and found the 'primer function' of RNA fragments attached to the DNA.

George Oliver

(1841–1915) British cardiologist who invented a hemacytometer, sphygmometer, wrote *Studies on Blood Pressure*, and studied the thyroid, thymus and pituitary glands.

Garcia da Orta

(1501–1568) Portuguese physician and skilful clinician, who wrote a materia medica based on his experiences in India, and described cholera and amoebic dysentery for the first time.

Sir William Osler

(1849–1919) Brilliant Canadian–British physician and polymath who wrote over 730 books and articles

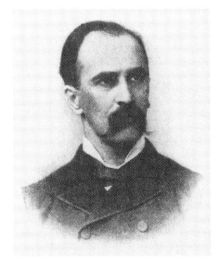

Sir William Osler

including *The Principles and Practice of Medicine*, studied blood platelets, polycythemia rubra vera, lupus erythematosus, treated Addison disease with adrenal extract, and studied exophthalmic goiter. He was a great advocate of patient-oriented scientific medicine.

John Conrad Otto

(1774–1844) American physician who gave the first definitive clinical description of hemophilia and used sodium sulfate in treatment, studied epilepsy, and used opium and calomel in the treatment of rheumatism.

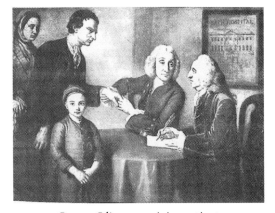

George Oliver examining patients

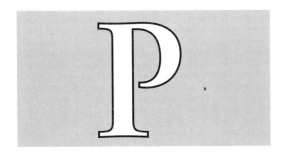

Antonio Pacchioni

(1665–1726) Italian anatomist who studied the structure and function of the dura mater, and described arachnoidal granulations (Pacchionian bodies) and depressions in the skull.

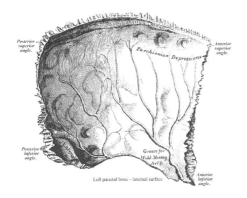

Pacchioni corpuscles

Sir James Paget

(1814–1899) British surgeon who gave the first description of osteitis deformans, and studied congenital pseudoarthritis and osteogenesis, and described an eczemoid cancerous lesion of the nipple.

George Emil Palade

(b 1912) Romanian cell biologist and Nobel laureate who developed cell fractionation and described the organelles within the cell, he also showed that protein synthesis occurs on the RNA strands and the proteins are then enclosed in vacuoles for transport out of the cell.

Richard De Forest Palmiter

(b 1942) American biochemist who produced the first transgenic mice, by injecting the human growth hormone gene into the mouse embryo, creating a vital tool for research of control mechanisms of gene expression.

Joseph Pancoast

(1805–1882) American physician and surgeon who developed new procedures for the treatment of cataract, tic douloureux, extrophy of the bladder, and thoracentesis for empyema.

George Nicholas Papanicolaou

(1883–1962) Greek-born American physiologist and microscopic anatomist who discovered changes in cells in the wall of the vagina during the estrus cycle. From this he went on to identify precancerous cells from cervical scrapings, and his cytological technique is now used in detection of cervical and other cancers (the Pap smear).

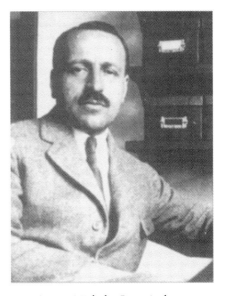

George Nicholas Papanicolaou

Alwin M Pappenheimer

(1878–1955) American hematologist who described iron granules in erythrocytes in peripheral blood, showed trench fever to be transmitted by lice, and used cod liver oil in treatment of rickets.

Paracelsus

(1493–1541) Swiss physician and alchemist, whose real name was Theophrastus von Hohenheim, who wrote on the nature and causes of diseases, and advocated simple remedies including opium, sulfur, mercury and lead.

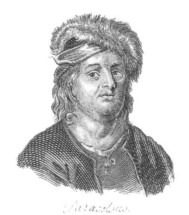

Paracelsus

Arthur Beck Pardee

(b 1921) American biochemist who worked on tumor metabolism, antibody reactions, discovered feedback control of amino acid synthesis, and investigated serum peptides.

Ambroise Paré

(1510–1590) Greatest French surgeon of the period who revolutionized treatment of gunshot wounds, described polyorchidism, varicocele, exophthalamic goiter, and epilepsy, developed braces and prostheses, devised an instrument to hold the teeth apart and used trephination.

Sir Alan Sterling Parkes

(1900–1990) British physician who studied endocrinology and reproduction and wrote *The Internal Secretions of the Ovary*, and *Patterns of Sexuality and Reproduction*.

James Parkinson

(1755–1824) British physician and paleontologist, remembered for his eponymous disease, paralysis agitans, who described the first case of appendicitis in which perforation was recognized as the cause of death, and also wrote on gout and gouty arthritis.

Caleb Hillier Parry

(1755–1822) British physician who presented the first recorded case of facial hemiatrophy, described congenital idiopathic dilatation of colon, and gave a complete account of exophthalmic goiter in *Enlargement of the Thyroid Gland in connection with Enlargement or Palpitation of the Heart*.

Louis Pasteur

(1822–1895) French chemist and father of bacteriology and the germ theory of disease, who introduced pasteurization to destroy pathogenic bacteria, and developed attenuated strains for vaccination.

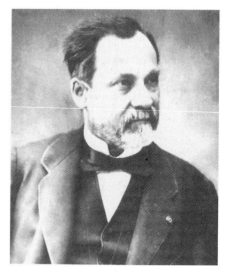

Louis Pasteur

Nicolas C Paulesco

(1869–1931) Romanian endocrinologist who used suprarenal extracts in treatment, studied the effects of thyroid removal, and isolated 'pancreine' (insulin).

Linus Carl Pauling

(1901–1994) American scientist and double Nobel laureate who wrote on the quantum mechanics of the chemical bond in *The Nature of the Chemical Bond*, studied protein structure, serological reactions, and the chemical basis of hereditary disease, advocated vitamin C to prevent infection, and worked for nuclear disarmament.

Friedrich Pauwels

(1885–1980) German orthopedic surgeon who worked on biomechanical influences on growth and behaviour of bone and cartilage.

Ivan P Pavlov

(1849–1936) Russian physiologist and Nobel laureate in 1904 for work on gastric secretions, he is remembered particularly for his research on conditioned reflexes, and wrote *Lectures on the work of the Digestive Glands*.

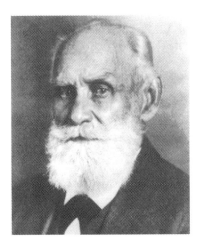

Ivan P Pavlov

Jean Pecquet

(1622–1674) French physician and anatomist who discovered the thoracic duct and receptaculum chyli.

Pierre Joseph Pelletier

(1788–1842) French chemist who studied alkaloids and their effects on humans, isolated strychnine, toluene, quinine and caffeine, and elucidated the ring structure of alkaloids.

Wilder Graves Penfield

(1891–1976) Canadian neurosurgeon whose research on the higher functions of the brain in animal experiments and in conscious surgical patients contributed to the understanding of speech and epilepsy.

Lionel Sharples Penrose

(1898–1972) British geneticist who carried out a major survey into the causes of mental illness, opposed attempts at eugenics, contributed to the understanding of Down syndrome, and gene mapping.

Candace Pert

(b 1946) American biochemist who studied the binding of synthetic opiates to specific brain receptor sites and identified some such sites, which suggested the existence of natural opiate substances in the brain.

Georg C Perthes

(1869–1927) German orthopedic surgeon who pioneered radiotherapy for malignant tumors, and described osteochondrosis of the proximal femoral epiphysis in children.

Max Ferdinand Perutz

(b 1914) Austrian-born British molecular biologist and Nobel laureate who studied the structure of hemoglobin using X-ray crystallography, its genetic variants, evolution, and binding to oxygen.

Sir Rudolf Albert Peters

(1889–1982) British biochemist who studied thiamine and its involvement in intermediary metabolism, and the organic binding of fluoride in bone.

Jean Louis Petit

(1674–1750) French surgeon and inventor of the screw tourniquet, who provided the first descriptions of softening of bones, studied formation of clots in wounded arteries, and performed the first mastoidectomy.

Johann Conrad Peyer

(1653–1712) Swiss anatomist who discovered Peyer patches, aggregates of lymphoid follicles in the submucosa and lamina propria of the terminal ileum, which are particularly affected in typhoid fever.

Richard FJ Pfeiffer

(1858–1945) German bacteriologist who discovered *Haemophilus influenzae* and (erroneously) suggested that it caused flu, observed the first complex immune factor, and discovered bacteriolysis.

Eduard FW Pflüger

(1829–1910) German physiologist who studied respiration and metabolism, and suggested that pancreatic diabetes was a nervous disorder.

Thomas Phayre

(c 1510–1560) British physician who wrote *The Regiment of Life* (1546), which contains *A Boke of Children*, the first UK contribution to pediatrics.

Philip Syng Physick

(1768–1837) Distinguished American surgeon who discovered the adsorbability of sutures made of animal tissue, and invented several surgical devices, including the forerunner of the modern guillotine for tonsillectomy.

Archangelus Piccolomineus

(1562–1605) Italian anatomist and early endo-crinologist who wrote *Anatomicae Praelectiones*, and described the suprarenal glands.

Sir George White Pickering

(1904–1980) British physician who studied hypertension and the involvement of peripheral resistance and hereditary factors, and later studied the mechanism of pain in peptic ulcers.

Gregory Goodwin Pincus

(1903–1967) American endocrinologist who studied steroid hormone effects on preventing mammalian

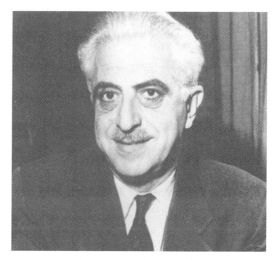

Gregory Goodwin Pincus

ovulation, and made fundamental contributions to the development of oral contraception.

Philippe Pinel

(1745–1826) French physician who was the first to treat the insane humanely, recording his methods in *Traité médico-philosophique sur l'aliénation mentale* in 1801.

Pierre Adolphe Piorry

(1794–1879) French physician and the inventor of the pleximeter, a pioneer of percussion, who wrote Traité sur la percussion médiate.

Nikolai Ivanovich Pirogoff

(1810–1881) Outstanding Russian military surgeon and pathologist who perfected a technique for sectioning frozen cadavers, was known for his amputation of the foot, introduced anesthesia to Russia and established a female nursing corps during the Crimean War.

Felix Platter

(1536–1614) Swiss physician and anatomist who wrote *Praxeos Medicinae*, described cretinism and goiter, hypertrophy of thymus as cause of infant death, studied psychiatric disorders, and was overseer of hospitals during plague outbreaks.

Pedro Ponce de Leon

(1520–1584) Spanish physician who wrote the first book on instruction for deaf-mutes.

Guido Pontecorvo

(b 1907) Italian-born British geneticist who proposed in the early 1950s that the gene is the unit of function in genetics.

Rodney Robert Porter

(1917–1985) British biochemist and Nobel laureate who developed a method of determining the N-terminus of a protein, and proposed the bilaterally symmetrical 4-chain structural basis of all immunoglobulins.

Pierre Carl Potain

(1825–1901) Outstanding French physician and cardiologist who invented an improved air sphygmomanometer, an aspirator for pleural effusion, described the Potain sign of dullness in right side of sternum in aortic dilatation, gallop rhythm, and jugular vein murmurs.

Percivall Pott

(1714–1788) British surgeon who wrote on *Tumors which Render the Bones Soft*, on the paralysis of

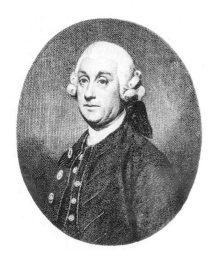

Percivall Pott

spinal tuberculosis (Pott paraplegia) a serious ankle injury (Pott fracture), and A *Treatise on Ruptures* which included an early description of congenital hernia, and a classic description of cancer of the scrotum and its treatment.

Sir John Pringle

(1707–1782) British founder of military medicine he advocated military hospitals as sanctuaries, the forerunner of the idea of the Red Cross, wrote *Observations on the Diseases of the Army*, including hygiene rules, and named influenza.

Georg Prochaska

(1749–1820) Czech physician and physiologist who discovered the olivary bodies, localized some cerebral functions, proposed a theory of sympathetic mechanism of gonad function, and was the first to describe reflex mechanisms of the nervous system.

William Prout

(1785–1850) British physician and physiological chemist who published an hypothesis of atomic weights, discovered hydrochloric acid in gastric juices, studied renal calculi and gravel in urine, and divided foodstuffs into fat, carbohydrate and protein constituents.

Stanley Ben Prusiner

(b 1942) American neurologist and Nobel laureate for his discovery of the disease-causing protein, the prion, responsible for the spongiform encephalo-pathies.

Mark Steven Ptashne

(b 1940) American molecular biologist who elucidated the actions of the lac repressor and operator of *E. coli* and the derepression of the operator gene in the presence of lactose, so improving our understanding of gene control and cell function.

Jan E Purkinje

(1787–1869) Czech physiologist who studied visual phenomena and the maintenance of balance. A

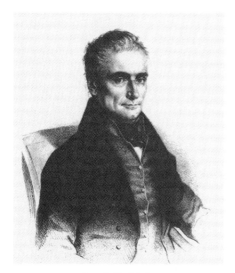

Jan E Purkinje

notable histologist, he described cells in the cerebellum and fibers in the myocardium

James Putnam

(1846–1918) American neurologist who studied neuritis from lead poisoning, polio, myxedema, spinal cord tumors, and subacute combined degeneration of the spinal cord.

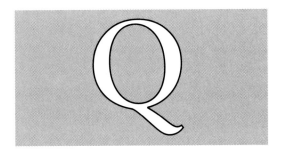

Juda Hirsch Quastel

(1899–1987) British biochemist who studied the biochemical aspects of brain function and mental disease, the effects of amphetamines and barbiturates, the synthesis of acetylcholine, and developed tests for schizophrenia.

Fritz de Quervain

(1868–1940) Swiss orthopedic surgeon and the first to make use of the medullary nail in a femur fracture, he described tendon sheath thickening, and a non-suppurtive form of thyroiditis.

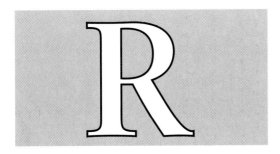

Bernadini Ramazzini

(1633–1714) Italian physician, epidemiologist and the founder of occupational medicine, who wrote *De morbis artificum diatriba*, the first systematic 'treatise on occupational disease', and studied cattle plague, malaria, and lathyrism.

Santiago Ramón y Cajal

(1852–1934) Spanish physician and neuroanatomist who studied the microstructure of the nervous system, brain, spinal cord and retina, proposed that information from dendrites is transmitted to axons of nerve cells, and Nobel laureate in 1906 for his studies on the brain.

François Ranchin

(1560–1641) French physician who described the diet, exercise and welfare, as well as the diseases of old age, he also wrote on surgery, pharmacology and the plague.

Louis A Ranvier

(1835–1922) French neurologist who discovered the Ranvier node, an area of localized constriction in the myelin sheath of nerve fibers, and studied the histology of nerves, and the lymph and circulation systems. In 1900 he proposed the concept of the reticuloendothelial system.

Pierre FO Rayer

(1793–1867) French physician who wrote several treatises and a classification of skin diseases, classic treatise on glanders and farcy (1837), a three-volume treatise on the kidney with an atlas, and on endemic hematuria.

Maurice Raynaud

(1834–1881) French physician remembered for his doctoral thesis *Local Asphyxia and Symmetrical Gangrene of the Extremities*, Raynaud syndrome.

Friedrich D von Recklinghausen

(1833–1910) German cardiologist and pathologist who described hemochromatosis, osteitis fibrosa cystica, multiple neurofibromatosis, adenomyosis of the uterus, and wrote on acromegaly, diabetes and the pancreas.

Peter Redfern

(1821–1912) British orthopedic surgeon and pathological anatomist who described the microscopic structure of normal and pathological cartilage.

Francesco Redi

(1626–1697) Italian physician and parasitologist who debunked the theory of spontaneous generation, and studied toxicology and snake venoms.

John Redman

(1722–1808) American physician, obstetrician and the first president of the College of Physicians of Philadelphia, he strongly advocated inoculation against smallpox, and described the management of the yellow fever epidemic of 1762.

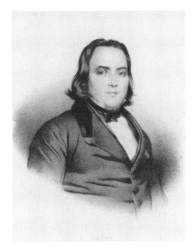

Pierre FO Rayer

Walter Reed

(1851–1902) American Army surgeon, involved in proving that yellow fever was transmitted by mosquitoes, he also showed that malaria was not caused by stagnant water.

Tadeus Reichstein

(1897–1996) Polish-born Swiss chemist and Nobel laureate who synthesized ascorbic acid, worked on the chemistry of the adrenal hormones, and isolated aldosterone.

Johann Christian Reil

(1759–1813) German physician who investigated the histology of the crystalline lens and discovered the island of Reil in the brain, he founded the first journal of psychiatry.

Hans Reiter

(1881–1969) German physician who studied spirochete diseases and described a sexually transmitted disease of non-specific urethritis, conjunctivitis and polyarthritis.

Ernst Remak

(1849–1911) German physician who described the Remak (femoral) reflex in spinal cord lesions, Remak paralysis in lead poisoning, and worked on peripheral nerves and neuropathies.

Robert Remak

(1815–1865) Brilliant German physician and anatomist who gave the first description of the axon cylinder and unmyelinated postganglionic axons of the sympathetic nervous system (Remak fibers), he was also a pioneer embryologist.

Henri Rendu

(1844–1902) Leading French physician of his day who described hereditary hemorrhagic telangiectasia, differentiating it from hemophilia.

Anders Adolf Retzius

(1796–1860) Swedish anatomist who identified the extraperitoneal cavity above the pubis – the cave of Retzius, and was an anthropologist who classified the human race on the basis of cranial measurements.

Rhazes

(850–932) Outstanding Persian physician who described diabetes mellitus, pregnancy, the sex organs, advised dietary regimes, first described and differentiated smallpox and measles, had some understanding of blood circulation, and wrote *Kitab El Hawi*, an encyclopedia of medicine.

Dickinson Woodruff Richards

(1895–1973) American physician and Nobel laureate who developed right heart catheterization for the study of blood pressure, oxygen tension and other variables, so increasing the understanding of shock and its treatment, and forming the basis of modern cardiology.

Benjamin Richardson

(1826–1896) British pharmacologist who studied the actions of amyl nitrite, and anesthetics, advanced the understanding of blood coagulation and wrote on the ill effects of alcohol.

Charles R Richet

(1850–1935) French physiologist and Nobel prizewinner who studied gastric secretion, and was a distinguished bacteriologist and statistician. He invented the term 'anaphylaxis'.

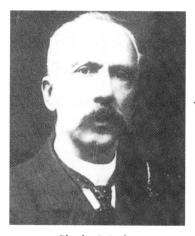

Charles R Richet

Sir Mark Henry Richmond

(b 1931) British molecular biologist who studied plasmid-mediated and transposon mediated resistance to antibiotics, and showed that resistance was most likely in hospitals with high antibiotic usage.

Philippe Ricord

(1799–1889) American physician and an authority on venereal diseases, who proved that syphilis and gonorrhea were separate diseases and divided syphilis into three stages.

Jean Riolan

(1580–1657) French physician and anatomist who described the seminiferous tubules, and introduced the term capsulae suprarenales for the adrenals.

Augustus Q Rivinus

(1652–1723) German anatomist who wrote a *Censura* classifying useless remedies, and ascribing most diseases to mites and minute worms.

Francesco Rizzoli

(1809–1880) Italian orthopedic surgeon who practiced osteotomy, devised an instrument for osteoclasis, and founded the famous orthopedic institute.

Frederick Chapman Robbins

(b 1916) American physiologist, pediatrician and Nobel laureate who developed a method of cultivating the polio virus that led to better methods of diagnosis and the development of a vaccine.

Richard Roberts

(b 1943) British molecular biologist and Nobel prizewinner who discovered that genes contains sections of DNA which carry no genetic information – introns.

Martin Rodbell

(1925–1998) American biochemist and Nobel laureate who discovered the G proteins, natural signal transducers in cellular communication that relay signals between a hormone receptor and the enzyme within a cell.

Roger of Palermo

(c 1170) Italian physician and surgeon who wrote *Practica chirurgiae*, the first European surgical text, and described treatment with seaweed or burned sponge and surgical treatment for goiter.

Karl von Rokitansky

(1804–1878) Outstanding Austrian pathologist who wrote *A Manual of Pathological Anatomy*, was the first to differentiate lobar from lobular pneumonia, gave the first description of spondylolisthesis, and described bacteria in lesions of malignant endocarditis.

Moritz H Romberg

(1795–1873) German neurologist who produced the first nosology of nervous system diseases, described ataxia in syphilis, achondroplasia, and facial hemiatrophy, now chiefly remembered for his classic sign of sensory ataxia.

Wilhelm C Röntgen

(1845–1923) German physicist and Nobel laureate who discovered the electromagnetic rays now known as X-rays.

Hendrik van Roonhuyze

(b 1625) Dutch surgeon who wrote *Heelkonstige Aanmerkkingen*, the first work on modern operative gynecology, advocated cesarean section, and was also an orthopedic surgeon, and noted for his operation for hare-lip.

William Cumming Rose

(1887–1984) American biochemist who studied the dietary importance of the 20 amino acids in proteins, and identified eight as essential for humans.

Nils Rosen von Rosenstein

(1706–1773) Swedish physician who wrote an important book on pediatrics, *Diseases of Children*, which includes an original implication of the kidneys in anasarca with bloody urine, a novel method of expelling worms, and gave detailed descriptions of smallpox, whooping cough and scarlet fever.

Eucharius Röslin

(d 1526) German obstetrician who wrote *Rosengarten*, an early book on obstetrics and midwifery, and revived podalic version.

Sir Ronald Ross

(1857–1932) British physician and Nobel laureate who found the malaria parasite in the mosquito stomach after they had bitten an infected patient, and worked out the malaria parasite life cycle in birds.

Francis Peyton Rous

(1879–1970) American pathologist who established the first blood banks, worked on cancer viruses (Rous sarcoma), and was a Nobel laureate in 1966.

Gustave Roussy

(1874–1948) Swiss neurologist who described thalamic syndrome, and wrote on spinal cord injuries and psychoneuroses.

Émile Roux

(1853–1933) French bacteriologist who worked on rabies and anthrax vaccines, developed treatment with antitoxin of diphtheria bacillus, and immunization with the toxin.

Wilhelm Roux

(1850–1924) German developmental embryologist who showed that germ plasm is passed intact from parent to offspring, thus suggesting a physical basis for heredity.

Gerald Mayer Rubin

(b 1950) American geneticist who produced the first transgenic fruit flies, which he used to study the regulation, activation and function of genes.

Olof Rudbeck

(1630–1702) Swedish physician who discovered the intestinal lymphatics and their connection to the thoracic duct.

Benjamin Rush

(1745–1813) One of the greatest American physicians, abolitionist and signatory to the Declaration of Independence, who described dengue fever, studied the effects of stimuli on excitability of the body, and epilepsy. He set up the first free dispensary in the US in 1786.

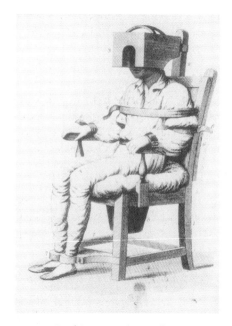

Rush's tranquilizing chair

Frederik Ruysch

(1638–1731) Dutch anatomist who discovered the valves in the lymphatics, devised techniques for visualization of blood vessels by injecting colored preservative into them, then describing the vascularity of the brain, heart and eye.

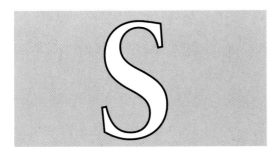

Albert Bruce Sabin

(1906–1993) Russian–American microbiologist who developed the first vaccine for dengue fever and Japanese B encephalitis, then worked on polio, developing the live attenuated oral vaccine that is now widely used.

Bernard Sachs

(1858–1944) American neurologist who worked on mental and nervous diseases, described infantile amaurotic familial idiocy (Tach–Sachs disease) and wrote *Nervous Diseases of Childhood* (1895).

Charles FM Saint

(1886–1973) British surgeon who wrote *An Introduction to Surgery* in 1925, his eponymous triad consists of hiatus hernia, cholelithiasis and diverticulosis of the colon.

Charles E Sajous

(1852–1928) American endocrinologist who wrote the first book in the US on internal secretions, and proposed the role of the adrenals in the body defense mechanisms.

Bert Sakmann

(b 1942) German electrophysiologist and Nobel prizewinner who helped to develop the patch–clamp method of recording electrical activity of a small area of membrane.

Guilielmo Salicetti

(c 1210–1277) Italian surgeon who wrote *Cyrurgia* containing the first mention of crepitus as a sign of fracture, described reduction of cervical dislocation, and distinguished between arterial and venous hemorrhage.

Jonas Edward Salk

(1914–1995) American immunologist who developed inactivated virus vaccine for polio.

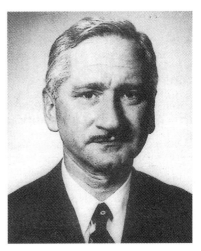

Jonas Edward Salk

Bengt Ingemar Samuelsson

(b 1934) Swedish biochemist and Nobel laureate who studied prostaglandin synthesis and metabolism, he showed that the E series lowers blood pressure and relaxes blood vessels while the F series has the opposite effect.

Sanctorius

(1561–1636) Italian physician who studied metabolism by measuring body weight, food intake, respiration, perspiration and excretion, he invented many instruments – including a weighing chair, a pendulum for measuring pulse rate, and a syringe for extracting bladder stones.

Ivar V. Sandström

(1852–1889) Swedish anatomist who discovered the parathyroid glands, recognizing them as distinct from lymph or accessory thyroid tissues.

Frederick Sanger

(b 1918) British biochemist and Nobel prizewinner who sequenced the amino acids in insulin, and then sequenced the bases of DNA of the virus Phi X 174 and the Epstein–Barr virus.

Nicolas Saucerotte

(1741–1814) French military surgeon and skilled neurosurgeon who established contralateral innervation, and described periodic coma and gigantism in acromegaly.

Ferdinand Sauerbruch

(1875–1951) German surgeon who refined thoracoplasty developed the negative pressure chamber for thoracic surgery.

Lewis Albert Sayre

(1820–1900) American orthopedic surgeon who invented the Sayre plaster jacket for Pott disease, and wrote *Spinal Disease and Spinal Curvature* (1877).

Antonio Scarpa

(c 1747–1832) Italian surgeon and brilliant anatomic illustrator who published on club foot in 1803, wrote on osteomyelitis and ophthalmology, and presented the first correct delineation of the nerves of the heart.

Andrew Victor Schally

(b 1926) Polish–American biochemist and Nobel laureate who isolated and analysed corticotrophin-releasing hormone, thrombotropin-releasing hormone, luteinizing hormone and somatostatin.

Fritz Richard Schaudinn

(1871–1906) German microbiologist who showed that amoebae were the cause of tropical dysentery and discovered *Entamoeba histolytica*. He also discovered *Spirochaeta pallida*, the cause of syphilis, and demonstrated that hookworm infection is contracted through the skin of the feet.

Carl W Scheele

(1742–1786) Great Swedish organic chemist who, in 1775, wrote his *Chemical Treatise on Air and Fire* that debunked the phlogiston theory, he also analysed urine and discovered uric acid.

Christoph Scheiner

(1575–1650) Austrian astronomer who wrote *Oculus*, described how images fall on the retina, changes in lens curvature, and accommodation of the eye.

Moritz Schiff

(1823–1896) German physician and physiologist who studied the action of the vagus nerve on the heart, the spinal pathways for pain and touch sensation, and the role of the thyroid gland.

Oswald Schmiedeberg

(1838–1921) German pharmacologist who wrote the standard book on the subject for his period, *Fundamentals of Pharmacology*, identified glycuronic acid, sinistrin and histozyme, studied the effects and value of digitalis and the effects of muscarine on the heart.

Rudolf Schoenheimer

(1894–1941) German-born American biochemist who used deuterium and heavy nitrogen to study the biochemical pathways of metabolism, showing that cycling of fats, protein and even bone undergoes continuous turnover, and distinguished pathways of saturated and unsaturated fatty acids.

Johann Lucas Schonlein

(1793–1864) Leading German clinician and proponent of scientific medicine who introduced the terms 'typhus abdominalis' and 'hemophilia' and gave the first descriptions of the metallic tinkle in pneumothorax and the auscultatory murmur over the femoral artery in aortic insufficiency. In 1837 he described peliosis rheumatica.

Arthur Schüller

(1874–1958) Austrian neurologist who developed the use of skull X-rays in the diagnosis of epilepsy, and described a disease caused by multiple histiocyteosis of bone.

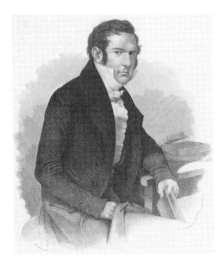

Johann Lucas Schonlein

Johann Schultes

(1595–1645) Renowned German surgeon and obstetrician who wrote an illustrated book on surgery that describes amputation of the breast, reduction of dislocation using the Scultetus bandage, and the use of forceps in delivery.

Theodor Schwann

(1810–1882) German physiologist who formulated cell theory, studied digestion, isolated pepsin, and discovered Schwann cells which surround peripheral nerve axons.

Hans Selye

(1907–1982) Canadian endocrinologist who developed the 'general adaptation syndrome' concept in 1936, linking stress and anxiety to disorders such as hypertension and rheumatic diseases, and wrote Textbook of Endocrinology.

Ignaz Philipp Semmelweis

(1818–1865) Hungarian obstetrician who studied puerperal fever, its causes and spread, and introduced strict hygiene measures to reduce mortality.

Jean-Baptiste Senac

(1693–1770) French cardiologist who studied respiration, wrote two volumes on heart disease and described pericarditis associated with pleurisy, and arteriosclerosis.

Servetus

(c 1511–1553) Spanish physician and theologian who was burned at the stake for suggesting that blood in the pulmonary circulation mixes with air from the lungs and passes through the heart – thus discovering the lesser circulation of the blood.

Baron Seutin

(1793–1865) Belgian orthopedic surgeon who devised a starch-impregnated linen bandage for immobilization of fractures that could be incised for inspection and then made rigid again.

Phillip Allen Sharp

(b 1944) American molecular biologist and Nobel laureate who invented S1 nuclease mapping for RNA, and discovered that genes are separated by DNA introns that do not contain genetic information.

Sir Edward Sharpey-Schäfer

(1850–1935) British physiologist who studied nerve regeneration and cerebral localization, effects of pituitary, the role of the pancreas in carbohydrate metabolism, postulated on the presence of a fluid he called 'insuline', and devised the prone-pressure method of artificial respiration.

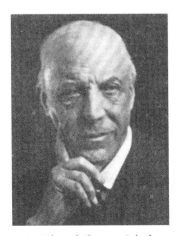

Sir Edward Sharpey-Schäfer

John Shaw

(1792–1827) British surgeon and anatomist who distinguished between rickets and other curvatures and advocated exercise in treatment.

Henry Clapp Sherman

(1875–1955) American biochemist who studied vitamin and mineral requirements in nutrition, established the daily requirement for calcium and its interaction with phosphorus and vitamin D, studied B vitamins in relation to polyneuritis, iron-deficiency anemia, and vitamin A requirements and storage.

Sir Charles S Sherrington

(1857–1952) British physiologist and Nobel laureate who discovered sensory receptors in muscles, joints and tendons, described proprioceptive sensation, and coined the term 'synapse'.

Sir John Simon

(1816–1904) British surgeon, pathologist and great public health reformer who suggested compulsory smallpox vaccination, and wrote an account of *English Sanitary Institutions*.

Sir James Young Simpson

(1811–1870) British obstetrician and pioneer of anesthesia in childbirth, used ether before he discovered the properties of chloroform, and was one of the founders of gynecology.

James Marion Sims

(1813–1883) Leading American gynecologist who developed the procedure for correction of vesicovaginal fistula, and designed the duckbill vaginal speculum, silver wire sutures and a double-curved silver indwelling catheter.

Joseph Skoda

(1805–1881) Austrian physician who correlated physical signs with pathological lesions, and described the drumlike sound heard on percussion of the chest above a pleural effusion.

William Smellie

(1697–1763) British obstetrician who introduced steel-lock, curved and double curved forceps, and wrote *Midwifery* the first book containing rules for the safe use of forceps.

Homer Smith

(1895–1962) American urologist who developed the use of inulin in kidney function tests to measure glomerular filtration rates.

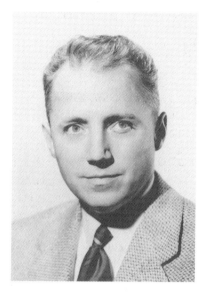

Homer Smith

Lester Smith

(1904–1992) British biochemist who developed commercial production of penicillins F, G and X using selective growth media, isolated vitamin B12 and showed that it contains cobalt, developed double-labeled vitamins for tracer studies, and developed an antibiotic complex active against streptococci, that had developed antibiotic resistance.

Michael Smith

(b 1932) British–Canadian biochemist and Nobel laureate who discovered site-specific mutagenesis, used to produce mutations at specific locations.

Nathan Smith

(1762–1829) Outstanding American physician, teacher and founder of medical schools in New England, he wrote on typhoid fever, ovarian tumor, and lithotomy, and performed staphyloplasty.

Theobald Smith

(1859–1934) American pioneer bacteriologist who implicated an insect vector (the tick) in Texas cattle fever, differentiated human from bovine strains of tubercle bacilli, and established techniques for examination of water, sewage and milk.

George Davis Snell

(1903–1996) American geneticist and Nobel prizewinner who was the first to show that X-rays can induce mutations in mammals, studied transplant rejection, and discovered the major histocompatibility complex (MHC).

John Snow

(1813–1858) Brilliant British anesthetist and epidemiologist who showed that cholera was spread through infected water, analyzed the relative merits of chloroform and ether and administered chloroform to Queen Victoria at the birth of two of her children.

Solomon Halbert Snyder

(b 1938) American psychiatrist and biochemist who studied brain biochemistry, catecholamines, ornithine decarboxylase, the effects of opiates and psychotropic drugs, enkephalins and endorphins and the effects of nitric oxide.

Samuel T von Soemmerring

(1755–1830) German neuroanatomist who wrote a monumental and accurate anatomy treatise, classified the cranial nerves, studied the brain, eye, ear, throat and nose, and described the injurious effects of corsets.

Soranus of Ephesus

(c 98–138) Greek physician who studied gynecology, obstetrics and pediatrics, he described podalic version, hysterectomy, and a vaginal speculum, and gave an early description of rickets.

Jean P Soulier

(b 1915) French hematologist who developed techniques to investigate blood coagulation, discovered anticoagulant – phenylindanedione, and described an autosomal, recessive syndrome of congenital bleeding.

Lazzaro Spallanzani

(1729–1799) Italian physiologist who refuted the theory of spontaneous generation, established that gastric juices and saliva were responsible for digestion, observed blood passing from arteries to veins, developed artificial insemination in dogs, and was the first to show that fertilization of an ovum required live sperm.

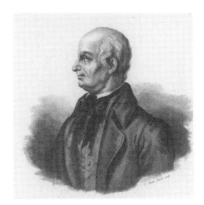

Lazzaro Spallanzani

Hans Spemann

(1869–1941) German embryologist and Nobel prizewinner who discovered the 'organizer function' of certain tissues during development, showing that embryonic cells are not pre-programed and that their differentiation is related to the tissues they are in contact with.

Roger W Sperry

(1913–1994) American neuroscientist and Nobel laureate who studied neural networks and proved they were independent of function, and worked on split-brain animals and humans showing the higher functions of the two hemispheres to be different.

Walter Spielmeyer

(1879–1935) German neurologist who studied juvenile amaurotic idiocy caused by lipid metabolism disturbance and, in 1911 wrote a book on microscopy of the nervous system.

Hu Ssu-Hui

(c 1330) Chinese physician who wrote *Yin Shan Cheng Yao*, detailing vitamin deficiency diseases, and a seaweed cure for goiter.

Roger Yate Stanier

(b 1916) Canadian biochemist who discovered the mandelate pathway, the mechanism of action of streptomycin, and studied tryptophan metabolism and bacterial pigments.

Wendell Meredith Stanley

(1904–1971) American virologist and Nobel laureate who isolated the tobacco mosaic virus, showed that it contained protein and nucleic acids, he went on to characterize it further, and noted that viruses can cause cancer.

Ernest H Starling

(1866–1927) Outstanding British physiologist who outlined his law of the heart: that the force of contraction of cardiac muscle is a function of the initial length of the muscle fibers. He wrote *Principles of Human Physiology* in 1912, discovered secretin, and studied lymph secretion.

William Howard Stein

(1911–1980) American biochemist and Nobel prizewinner who developed techniques for amino acid analysis, determined the bovine pancreatic ribonuclease amino acid structure, and first showed the phenomenon of convergent evolution in the plant protease papain and a protease from streptococcus.

Eugen Steinach

(1861–1944) Austrian physician who postulated the 'puberty' gland, and introduced the operation of ligature of the vas deferens for (transient!) rejuvenation.

Arthur Steindler

(1878–1959) American orthopedic surgeon and a pioneer of biomechanics, who wrote Orthopedic Operations in 1943.

Niels Stensen

(1638–1686) Danish anatomist who probably coined the term ovary in *Ova Viviparorum*, discovered the parotid (Stensen) duct, showed that muscle contraction could occur in an isolated muscle, and that its power was related to the sum of the fibrils.

Patrick Christopher Steptoe

(1913–1988) British gynecologist and reproductive biologist, who developed laparoscopy and pioneered *in vitro* fertilization and implantation of the human embryo.

George Miller Sternberg

(1838–1915) American military surgeon, bacteriologist and epidemiologist, responsible for the Yellow Fever Commission, who wrote *A Manual of Bacteriology, Infection and Immunity and Malaria and Malarial Diseases*. He isolated the pneumococcus (in the same year as Pasteur), and promoted the establishment of a nursing corps.

Nettie Maria Stevens

(1861–1912) American biologist who showed that sex is determined by particular chromosomes, and demonstrated the pairing of chromosomes in mosquitoes and flies.

Alfred Stillé

(1813–1900) American physician who prepared the first general pathology textbook in the US, a treatise on therapeutics and materia medica, was a founder of the American Medical Association and advocated the acceptance of women into medical schools.

Charles R Stockard

(1879–1939) American biologist and anatomist who worked on the estrous cycle, embryonic development and the chemical factors governing differentiation, regeneration, and growth.

Anton Stoerck

(1731–1803) Austrian physician who promoted emetics, investigated hemlock, stramonium, aconite, colchicum, pulsatilla, and hyoscyamus.

William Stokes

(1804–1878) Irish physician who reported the first case of cholera in the Dublin epidemic of 1832, and described diseases of the chest, the heart and aorta, and Cheyne-Stokes breathing. He wrote *Diseases of the Heart* (1854), and described the effect of an enlarged thyroid on heart action, arteries and the eye.

Marie C Stopes

(1880–1958) British endocrinologist and pioneer of birth control, who wrote about sex and contraception in *Married Love* in 1918.

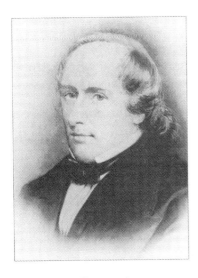

William Stokes

Solomon Stricker

(1834–1898) German physician who showed that sodium salicylate arrests rheumatic fever.

Georg FL Stromeyer

(1804–1876) German surgeon who Introduced tenotomy for club-foot, and wrote a book on operative orthopedics.

Adolph von Strümpell

(1853–1925) Russian-born German neurologist who described Marie–Strümpell disease (spondylitis deformans), Westphal–Strümpell disease (pseudosclerosis) and Strümpell disease or acute polioencephalitis.

Alfred Henry Sturtevant

(1891–1970) American geneticist who studied genetic crossing-over and recombination, made the first map of fruit fly chromosomes, and established mathematical principles for gene mapping.

James Batcheller Sumner

(1887–1955) American biochemist and Nobel laureate who was the first to crystalize an enzyme (urease) and show it to be a protein, later creating antibodies to it. He discovered and purified many other enzymes including monoamine oxidase.

Susruta

(c 800 BC) Famous Indian physician and surgeon who described surgery and bones in the body and left many authoritative books.

Johann Peter Süssmilch

(1707–1777) German scientist who combined vital and medical statistics and insisted on their moral and political significance, in his theological work, *The Divine Ordinance manifested in the Human Race through Birth, Death and Propagation*, a watershed in the study of population statistics..

Earl Wilbur Sutherland Jr

(1915–1974) American biochemist and Nobel

prizewinner who studied conversion of glycogen to glucose and the involvement of cyclic-AMP, so discovering the second messenger theory of hormone action.

Jan Swammerdam

(1637–1680) Dutch microscopist and outstanding natural scientist who described red blood corpuscles, discovered lymphatic valves, and mammalian ovarian follicles, and showed that fetal lungs float after respiration, and that muscle contraction occurs by stimulating the nerves.

Emanuel Swedenborg

(1688–1772) Swedish scientist and mystic who wrote a four-volume treatise on the brain in which he recognized the existence of the motor cortex, and the significance of the pituitary gland and postulated the neuron theory.

Gerhard van Swieten

(1700–1772) Austrian army physician, who wrote on hygiene, noted aura in hydrophobia in 1771, described symmetric gangrene in spinal affections, and used corrosive sublimate in syphilis.

Thomas Sydenham

(1624–1689) Outstanding British physician who was described as an 'Excellent Practical Physician' and a founder of modern clinical medicine, he described gout, rheumatic disorders, the effects of scurvy on joints, Sydenham chorea and hysteria, and regarded disease as a developmental process.

Franciscus Sylvius (de le Boë)

(1614–1672) Dutch physician, anatomist and founder of the iatrochemical school, who studied chemical imbalances in the blood, and discovered the Sylvian aqueduct connecting the third and fourth ventricles of the brain, in 1641.

Jacobus Sylvius

(1478–1555) French anatomist, teacher of Vesalius and Servetus, who proposed a system of identifying skeletal muscles, and another for vessels to which

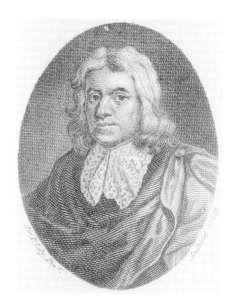

Thomas Sydenham

he gave the names 'jugular', 'femoral', 'renal' and 'popliteal'. He also gave the first description of the valve of the inferior vena cava.

James Syme

(1799–1870) Skilled British surgeon who wrote *Treatise on the excision of diseased joints* that described joint pathology and the ability of the periosteum to form osseous tissue. He was an early proponent of anesthesia and devised an amputation through the ankle joint.

Richard Laurence Millington Synge

(b 1914) British biochemist and Nobel laureate who was involved in development of modern chromatography techniques for analysis of biological molecules.

Albert von Szent-Györgyi

(1893–1986) Born in Hungary and emigrated to the US where he discovered vitamin C in the adrenal cortex, crystallized vitamins C and B2, and studied muscle contraction and myosin inhibition and cleavage. He was awarded the Nobel Prize in 1937.

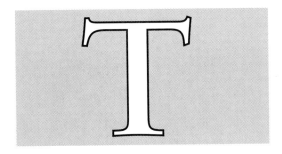

Gasparo Tagliacozzi

(1546–1599) Italian surgeon who performed facial reconstruction and rhinoplasty, specializing in surgical correction of deformities. Though reviled by his peers, and condemned by the church, he is considered the father of plastic surgery.

Edward Lawrie Tatum

(1909–1975) American geneticist and Nobel laureate who formulated the one gene one enzyme hypothesis and demonstrated the role of genes in metabolism using mutants of the mold Neurospora.

Helen Brooke Taussig

(1898–1986) American pediatrician who with Alfred Blalock, pioneered 'blue baby' operations, creating a new specialty in pediatric cardiac surgery.

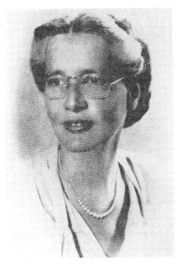

Helen Brooke Taussig

Charles Fayette Taylor

(1827–1899) American orthopedic surgeon who introduced remedial exercises, advocating them for many conditions, and developed a brace for Pott disease.

Howard Martin Temin

(1934–1994) American virologist and Nobel laureate who formulated the provirus hypothesis of the copying of viral DNA into the host cell DNA. He isolated reverse transcriptase from retroviruses, now widely used in genetic engineering.

James Thacher

(1754–1844) American physician and prolific writer whose *American Modern Practice: or, a Simple Method of Prevention and Cure of Diseases* contains an important introductory section on the history of the 17 medical schools then in the Colonies. He also wrote the first *American Medical Biography*.

Max Theiler

(1899–1972) South African-born American virologist and Nobel prizewinner who showed that yellow fever was caused by a filterable virus, attenuated a strain of the virus, and developed the 17-D vaccine suitable for large-scale immunization.

Theophrastus

(c 372–287 BC) Famous Greek physician and philosopher who studied pain and recorded that two drachms of strychnos produced delusions, three insanity, and four death.

Hugo Teodor Theorell

(1903–1982) Swedish biochemist and Nobel laureate who crystallized and determined the molecular weight of myoglobin, studied riboflavin (vitamin B2) and cytochrome C, purified diphtheria antitoxin and introduced electrophoresis and fluorescence spectroscopy.

Donnall Thomas

(b 1920) American hematologist and Nobel prizewinner who studied bone marrow transplantation, and used tissue typing techniques and immunosuppressive drugs to enable bone marrow transplants in the treatment of aplastic anemia, leukemia and some genetic diseases.

Hugh Owen Thomas

(1834–1891) Founder of British orthopedics, who wrote *Principles of Treatment of Diseased Joints* and other books, and developed prostheses and splints, including Thomas splints for the hip and knee.

Robert AA Tigerstedt

(1853–1923) Finnish endocrinologist who studied the effect of the kidneys on circulation, discovered renin, and used it in experiments with nephrectomized animals.

Simon-André Tissot

(1728–1797) Swiss physician who promoted variolation for protection against smallpox, wrote on epilepsy, nervous diseases and hygiene, and wrote *Avis au peuple sur la santé* (1760).

Alexander Robertus Todd

(b 1907) British medical chemist and Nobel laureate who worked on the structure and synthesis of the four DNA bases and the attachment to these of sugar and phosphate molecules to form nucleotides.

Susumu Tonegawa

(b 1939) Japanese molecular biologist and Nobel prizewinner who used restriction enzymes and recombinant DNA to study and elucidate mechanisms of antibody diversity where the genes undergo changes enabling them to make a range of new antibodies.

Francesco Torti

(1658–1741) Italian physician who wrote a book on intermittent fevers, named malaria, and used cinchona bark (quinine) as treatment.

George Gilles de la Tourette

(1857–1904) French neurologist who described a syndrome of violent muscle jerks of face, shoulders

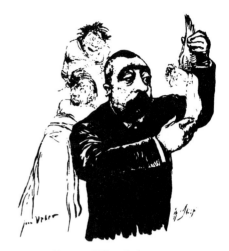

George Gilles de la Tourette

and extremities, and also worked on hysteria and hypnotism.

Ludwig Traube

(1818–1876) Outstanding German physician and pathologist who, in 1856, published a monograph on the association between ventricular hypertrophy and renal lesions, described hypertension, pulsus alternans, the pathology of fevers, and the use of digitalis in heart disease.

Benjamin Travers

(1783–1858) British surgeon and anatomist who wrote an excellent systematic monograph on the eye, he was the first surgeon in England to specialize in surgery of the eye.

Friedrich Trendelenburg

(1844–1924) German surgeon who described a test for competence of the long saphenous vein, instability of the hip from dislocation (Trendelenburg sign), vesicovaginal fistula, varicose veins, thrombophlebitis, and bone and joint injuries. He was the first to perform gastrostomy and to operate for pulmonary embolism.

Sir Frederick Treves

(1853–1923) British surgeon who studied peritonitis and intestinal obstruction, improved the operation

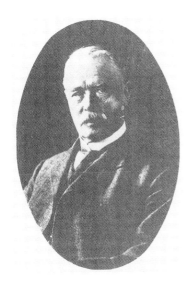

Friedrich Trendelenburg

for appendicitis, and wrote on the *Elephant Man and Other Reminiscences*, about his patient, Carey Merrick, a sufferer from neurofibromatosis.

Gottfried Reinhold Treviranus

(1776–1837) German anatomist, physiologist and botanist who introduced the concept of 'biology', and was famous for his study of the louse.

Théodore Tronchin

(1709–1781) Swiss physician who wrote *De colica Pictonum* showing that Poitou colic was caused by lead poisoning, he was a pioneer of inoculation, psychotherapy, and advocated suspension in spinal curvature.

Armand Trousseau

(1801–1867) Outstanding French clinician who led the renaissance of French medicine, he was the first to perform tracheotomy for the relief of croup, and described the spasm of latent tetany.

Joseph Trueta

(1897–1977) Spanish orthopedic and military surgeon and one of the first to treat osteomyelitis with penicillin, who also established standards for war surgery.

Hugh Compson Trumble

(1894–1962) Australian orthopedic surgeon who developed extra-articular bone graft arthrodesis of the hip joint in 1932.

Nicolaas Tulp

(1593–1674) Dutch anatomist and physician and subject of Rembrant's painting 'The Anatomy Lesson', who wrote a book which included details of a left-side head injury causing contralateral paralysis, treatment of carcinoma of the bladder, and a clinical description of beriberi.

Daniel Turner

(1667–1740) British physician, recipient of the first diploma granted by an American school and the founder of dermatology, who wrote *De Morbis Cutaneis*, and introduced calamine ointment (Turner cerate) into treatment.

Frederick William Twort

(1877–1950) British pioneer bacteriologist who studied acid-fast bacteria, isolated vitamin K from tubercle bacteria, and discovered the bacteriophage in 1915 calling it 'transmissible lytic agent'.

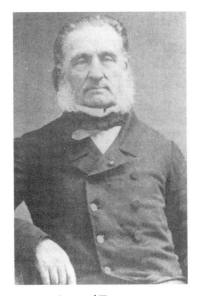

Armand Trousseau

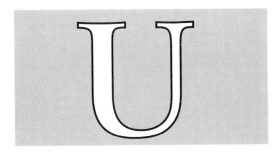

Paul Gerson Unna

(1850–1929) Leading German dermatologist who developed staining techniques, described seborrhoeic eczema, founded a journal of practical dermatology, and wrote *Histopathology of the Skin*.

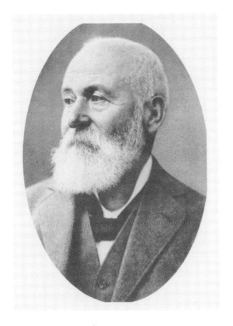

Paul Gerson Unna

Johann August Unzer

(1727–1799) German neurologist who distinguished voluntary from involuntary movements, and described conditional (Pavlovian) reflexes.

Erich Urbach

(1893–1946) Austrian clinical dermatologist and proponent of the allergic pathogenesis of skin disorders, who described familial lipoproteosis and necrobiosis lipoidica diabeticorum.

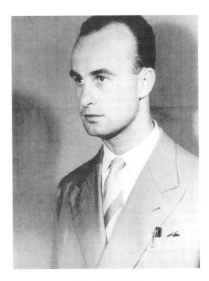

Erich Urbach

Hans Henrikson Ussing

(1911–1997) Danish biophysicist who studied mechanisms of active and passive transport across biological membranes using deuterium isotope, and proposed cyclical carrier systems of permeability.

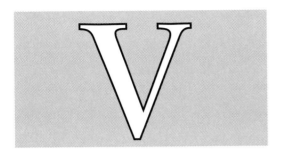

Gabriel Gustav Valentin

(1810–1883) German experimental physiologist who studied the nerve ganglia, embryology, and identified myoglobin in muscles, and ciliary epithelial motion.

Antonio Maria Valsalva

(1666–1723) Italian anatomist and physiologist, who wrote an outstanding book on the anatomy of the human ear, and invented his well known maneuver for relieving obstructions from the Eustachian tubes.

Sir John Robert Vane

(b 1927) British pharmacologist and Nobel laureate who studied adrenergic receptors and the role of the lung in drug uptake and metabolism, and investigated prostaglandin chemistry and the pain relieving properties of aspirin.

Harold E Varmus

(b 1939) American molecular biologist and Nobel laureate in 1989, for his discovery of oncogenes, fundamental to the understanding of cancer mechanisms.

Costanzo Varolio

(1543–1575) Italian anatomist who investigated the nervous system, describing the crura cerebri and pons, and also the ileocecal valve.

Alfred Velpeau

(1795–1867) French surgeon who wrote comprehensive treatises on midwifery, surgical anatomy and operative surgery, developed the Velpeau bandage and described the Velpeau (inguinal) hernia.

Jean André Venel

(1740–1791) Swiss orthopedic surgeon, considered the father of orthopedics, who founded the first orthopedic institute in the world, and stressed the benefit of sunlight in treatment.

Andreas Vesalius

(1514–1564) Outstanding Belgian anatomist and surgeon who wrote *De Humani Corporis Fabrica*, and described the thyroid, pituitary and thalamus, and the ovaries.

Raymond de Vieussens

(1641–1715) French physician and anatomist who studied the brain and spinal cord, describing the cerebellum, the white matter of the cerebrum, and the structure of the ear, and was the first to describe aortic incompetence and mitral stenosis.

Vincent du Vigneaud

(1901–1978) American biochemist who studied amino acid chemistry and metabolism, including the roles of choline, lecithin and methionine, showed the importance of thiamine in nutrition, and synthesized thiamine, penicillin, vasopressin and oxytocin.

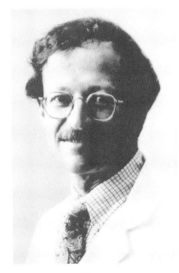

Harold E Varmus

Arnold of Villanova

(c1235–1311) Italian physician who wrote on goiter and treatment with seaweed and burned sponge, and discovered the poisonous nature of carbon monoxide and of decayed meat.

Jean-Antoine Villemin

(1827–1892) French physician who made the fundamental discovery that material taken from a tuberculous lung and inoculated into an animal produced the disease, pointing to the existence of an infective agent.

Rudolf Virchow

(1821–1902) German founder of cellular pathology, who regarded disease as a cellular response to change, studied parasites, leukemia, inflammation, thrombosis, public health, uncalcified bone in rickets, spina bifida occulta, intervertebral disc prolapse, and atherosclerotic lesions.

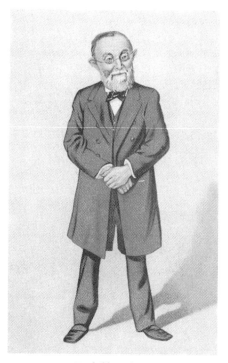

Rudolf Virchow

Artturi Ilmari Virtanen

(1895–1973) Finnish biochemist and Nobel prizewinner who studied bacterial carbohydrate metabolism and proteases, and isolated hemoglobin.

Cecile Vogt

(1875–1962) French neurologist who did early work on the neuroanatomy of the thalamus, studied hereditary pseudobulbar palsy and congenital chorea, and mapped the brain.

Peter Vogt

(b 1932) German-born US virologist who studied the relationship between oncogenes and retroviruses and showed that there are two ways the retrovirus can affect the gene and lead to carcinogenesis.

Karl von Voit

(1831–1908) German physiologist who studied nutrition and metabolism, showing that carbohydrate was converted to fat, he developed the Voit Law of nitrogen metabolism, studied leukemia and diabetes, and showed that heat given off by a body was related to metabolic activity.

Richard von Volkmann

(1830–1889) German surgeon who showed that arterial occlusions cause ischemic muscle paralysis and contractures, and was the first surgeon to excise the rectum for tumor.

Alessandro Volta

(1745–1827) Italian orthopedic surgeon who differentiated efferent and afferent nerve action in muscles, and showed repeated electrical stimulation of muscle can cause tetanic contraction.

Serge Voronoff

(1866–1951) Russian-born French physiologist and surgeon who studied aging and grafted monkey testicular glands into humans to restore potency, and monkey thyroid into backward children in an attempt to make them normal (unsuccessfully).

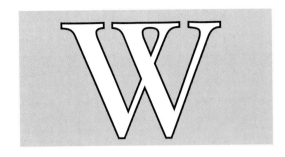

Conrad Hal Waddington

(1905–1975) British embryologist and geneticist who studied epigenesis and effects of chemical messengers and environmental influences on embryonic cell development and differentiation.

Julius Wagner-Jauregg

(1857–1940) Austrian neurologist, psychiatrist and Nobel laureate who developed fever therapy for mental disease, using malarial inoculation in general paralysis, a late stage of syphilis.

Thomas Wakley

(1795–1862) Controversial British surgeon, reformer and the founder of *The Lancet* in 1823, which published reports of hospital lectures and operations, he also published details of quack medicines and failures by surgeons whom he called 'Bats and Corruptionists'.

Selman Abraham Waksman

(1888–1973) Russian-born American microbiologist and Nobel prizewinner who isolated antibacterial substances from soil actinomycetes, discovered the anticancer drug actinomycin, the first effective anti-TB drug streptomycin, and neomycin.

George Wald

(1906–1997) American biochemist and Nobel laureate who studied the retinal pigment visual purple (rhodopsin) and its conversion by light to vitamin A, and established the relationship between vitamin A, night blindness, and vitamin-deficient retinopathy.

Wilhelm Waldeyer-Hartz

(1839–1921) German comparative anatomist and histologist who classified cancers according to their embryological cell origin: carcinomas from epithelial cells, and sarcomas from connective tissue.

Augustus Desire Waller

(1856–1922) British physiologist and founder of electrocardiography, who showed that currents established by the beat of the heart could be recorded on the skin, and also studied nerve excitation and the physiology of general anesthesia.

Augustus Volney Waller

(1816–1870) British physiologist who studied the nervous system, discovering Wallerian degeneration of the myelin sheath after section of nerve fibers, and studied vasoconstrictor properties of sympathetic nerves and dilation of the iris in response to light.

Otto Heinrich Warburg

(1883–1970) German biochemist and Nobel prizewinner who discovered the important role of iron in cells, developed the gas manometer, and studied the metabolism of cancer cells.

John Collins Warren

(1778–1856) American surgeon who, in 1846, used

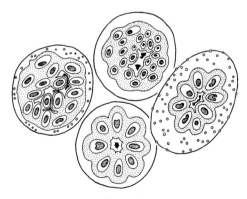

Bacteria

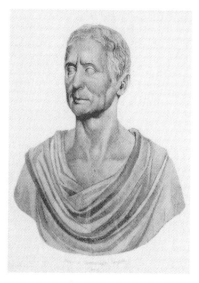

John Collins Warren

ether as an anesthetic in surgery for a tumor of the neck, he also operated on a natural fissure of the soft palate, and was a founder of the *New England Journal of Medicine and Surgery*.

Robert Wartenberg

(1887–1956) American neurologist who described Wartenberg paresthetic neuralgia of the hand.

August Paul von Wassermann

(1866–1925) German bacteriologist who discovered his eponymous serological test for syphilis, studied complement fixation and, later, cancer chemotherapy.

Benjamin Waterhouse

(1754–1846) American physician who introduced Jenner's method of cowpox vaccination against smallpox into the US, and was the first professor of medicine at Harvard.

James Dewey Watson

(b 1928) American molecular biologist and Nobel laureate who worked on the elucidation of the structure of DNA, and wrote a personal account in The Double Helix, and the textbook *Molecular Biology of the Gene*.

Sir Thomas Watson

(1792–1882) British physician who wrote the first treatise on practice of medicine, *Lectures on the Principles and Practice of Physic*, in 1843, which remained the principal English textbook of medicine for over 30 years.

Sir David John Weatherall

(b 1933) British physician who studied the genetic aspects, prenatal diagnosis and clinical outcome of thalassemias.

Ernst Heinrich Weber

(1795–1878) German anatomist and physiologist who studied digestion and showed it to be involved with glandular secretions, devised a quantitative test for measuring the sensory 'threshold' of the skin, and demonstrated the inhibitory effect of vagal stimulation.

Carl Weigert

(1845–1904) German pathologist who developed staining of tissues with aniline dyes, devised the Weigert stain for myelin sheaths, and stains for fibrin, neuroglia and elastic fibers, studied tissue response to insult and repair in smallpox, and classified glomerular nephritis.

Robert Allan Weinberg

(b 1942) American biochemist who studied the causes of cancer, such as the acquisition of cancer-susceptible genes or loss of tumor suppressor genes, and elucidated the role of the Rb1 suppressor gene in a rare childhood retinal cancer.

August FL Weisman

(1834–1914) German biologist who developed the theory that the information required for the make-up of the final form of an organism is present within the germ cells. He also realised that reduction division must occur to prevent doubling of the genetic material on each generation.

Robin Weiss

(b 1940) British molecular biologist who studied the role of retroviruses in cancers, and the mechanism of HIV entry into cells.

N. Charles Weissman

(b 1931) Swiss molecular biologist who identified the DNA sequences recognized by RNA polymerase in transcription for the high level of expression of genes, and worked on the structure, function and cloning of insulin genes, important in the advance of the treatment of diabetes.

William Henry Welch

(1850–1934) American bacteriologist and pathologist who studied diphtheria toxin, and identified the first anerobic organism, the cause of gas gangrene: *Clostridium welchii*.

Thomas Huckle Weller

(b 1915) American virologist and Nobel laureate who developed techniques for cultivation of the polio virus, isolated the causative agent of chickenpox and shingles, and identified the cytomegalovirus.

William Charles Wells

(1757–1817) American physician who detected albumin in urine in anascara, hematuria and albuminuria in scarlet fever and dropsy, described cardiac complications in rheumatic fever, and studied the mechanism of the eye.

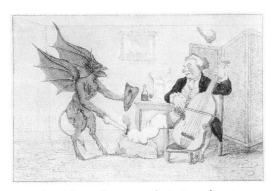

An eighteenth century depiction of gout

Johann Jakob Wepfer

(1620–1695) Swiss anatomist and physician who described hemorrhagic extravasations in the cerebrum in apoplexy, subdural hematoma, and duodenal glands and studied poisons.

Paul Gottlieb Werlhof

(1699–1767) German physician who gave an original description of purpura hemorrhagica (idiopathic thrombocytopenic purpura) in 1775.

Karl Wernicke

(1848–1905) German neuropsychiatrist who described sensory aphasia and Wernicke encephalopathy of ophthalmoplegia, nystagmus and cerebellar ataxia with tremors (associated with amnesia and confabulation), caused by thiamine deficiency.

Thomas Wharton

(1614–1673) British physician who wrote *Adenographia: sive glandularum totius corporis descriptio*, describing the lymphatic glands, pancreas, thymus, salivary glands, thyroid, pituitary, testicles, and ovaries, and his name was given to the submaxillary salivary duct.

George Hoyt Whipple

(1878–1976) American pathologist and Nobel laureate who studied hemoglobin and anemia, and produced a liver extract for the treatment of pernicious anemia. He described a chronic inflammatory disease of the bowel which bears his name.

Daniel Whistler

(1619–1684) British physician who wrote the earliest comprehensive account of the symptoms of a disease in *The Rickets*.

Charles White

(1728–1813) British surgeon and pioneer in aseptic midwifery, who was the first to excise the head of the humerus, and described painful 'white leg' in the puererium.

Robert Whytt

(1714–1766) Physician and foremost British neurologist of his time, who showed that the integrity of the whole spinal cord was not necessary for reflex action, discovered spinal shock, described tubercular meningitis in children, and wrote an essay *On the Vital and other Involuntary Motions of Animals* in 1751.

Georges Fernand Widal

(1862–1929) Algerian-born French physician and bacteriologist who developed the diagnostic agglutination test for typhoid fever, attributed edema to retention of sodium chloride, and studied anaphylaxis and hemolytic anemias.

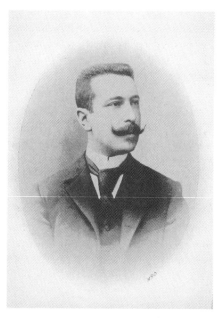

Georges Fernand Widal

Eric F Wieschaus

(b 1947) American developmental biologist and Nobel laureate for his work on the genetic controls of early embryonic development, showing that there were three sets of genes involved in control mechanisms.

Torsten Nils Wiesel

(b 1924) Swedish neurobiologist and Nobel prizewinner who studied processing of visual information by the brain, discovering the hierarchical pathway of processing by nerve cells from the retina to the cerebral cortex, that proved useful in treatment of children with sight impairment.

Samuel Wilks

(1824–1911) British physician and anatomist who gave the definitive description of Addison disease, reported on treatment of epilepsy with bromide, described the visceral effects of syphilis (including aortic aneurysm), and was the first to describe bacterial endocarditis and myasthenia gravis.

Robert Willan

(1757–1812) British physician and a founder of modern dermatology, who described eczema and lupus, divided cutaneous diseases into eight classes, and established nomenclature in his great work *The description and treatment of cutaneous diseases*.

De Forest Willard

(1846–1910) American orthopedic and pediatric surgeon, a pioneer in nerve grafting and suture, who advocated Listerism (antisepsis).

Thomas Willis

(1621–1675) British physician and anatomist who described the pineal body, the influence of the glands in the uterus and testes, the pathology and clinical features of diabetes, the Circle of Willis of the brain, and introduced the term 'neurologie'.

Max Wilms

(1867–1918) German surgeon who studied tumors of the kidney and the ovary, and described nephroblastoma (Wilms tumor).

Edmund Beecher Wilson

(1856–1939) American founder of modern genetics, who wrote *The Cell in Development and Inheritance*, demonstrated the importance of sex chromosomes

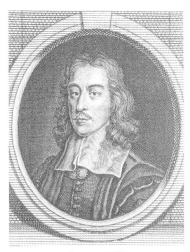

Thomas Willis

in heredity and the significance of cells as the building blocks of life.

SA Kinnier Wilson

(1877–1937) Brilliant American-born British neurologist who described a rare disease comprising cerebral degeneration associated with cirrhosis of the liver (Wilson disease).

Philip D Wilson

(1886–1969) American orthopedic surgeon who developed the posterior capsuloplast for flexion contracture of knee, and wrote *Fractures and Dislocations* (1925).

Jakob Benignus Winslow

(1669–1760) Danish anatomist who wrote a the standard anatomy textbook, *Exposition anatomique de la structure du corps humain* in 1733, the classic work for over 100 years, and described the formanen between the greater and lesser peritoneal sacs.

Thomas M Winterbottom

(1765–1859) British physician who gave one of the first descriptions of African sleeping sickness in his book on health and diseases of native Africans.

Maxwell M Wintrobe

(1901–1986) Canadian-born US hematologist who studied anemia and nutritional and vitamin deficiencies, devised the hematocrit tube, and wrote a classic textbook on hematology.

Johann Georg Wirsung

(1600–1643) German anatomist who discovered the pancreatic duct in 1642.

Richard Wiseman

(1622–1676) British surgeon who wrote *Severall Chirugicall Treatises* in 1676, a treatise on gonorrhea, and first described the 'white swellings' of tuberculosis of the joints.

Caspar Wistar

(1761–1818) American physician and anatomist who wrote the first comprehensive text on anatomy in the US, *A System of Anatomy for the Use of Students of Medicine* in 1811.

William Withering

(1741–1799) British physician and botanist who described the epidemics of scarlatina, recommended treatment for phthisis, and was the first to use foxglove in treatment of dropsy.

Julius Wolff

(1836–1902) German orthopedic surgeon who developed thin bone sectioning, and wrote *The Law of Bone Transformation*, relating structure and shape of bone development to external forces and change in function.

Kaspar F Wolff

(1733–1794) German pioneer in embryology and proponent of the germ-layer theory of embryonic organ development from blastodermic layers. Several embryonic structures are named after him.

Sir Christopher Wren

(1632–1713) British physician and architect who administered the first morphine injection (to a dog) thus paving the way for later transfusion, provided line drawings for Thomas Willis, and designed an artificial eye.

Sir Almroth Edward Wright

(1861–1947) British bacteriologist who developed a typhoid vaccine, studied parasitic diseases, and researched the protective power of blood against bacterial invasion.

Sewall Wright

(1889–1988) American geneticist who developed a mathematical model of evolution and showed that gene loss in isolated populations allows evolution to occur without natural selection – the Sewall Wright effect.

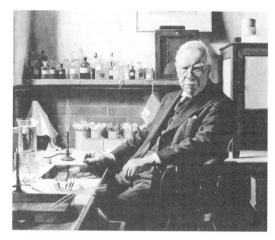

Sir Almroth Edward Wright

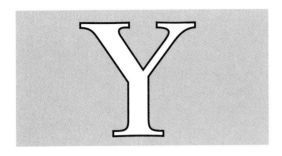

Rosalyn Yalow

(b 1921) American biophysicist and Nobel laureate who developed the radioimmunoassay for use in diabetes research and showed that anti-insulin antibodies are formed in adult diabetes, slowing clearance of labeled insulin. She also used RIA to study dwarfism, neurotransmitters and leukemia.

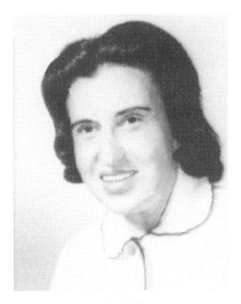

Rosalyn Yalow

Charles Yanofsky

(b 1925) American geneticist who showed that the sequences of bases in DNA determine the order of amino acids in proteins, and discovered the process of attenuation whereby production levels of an enzyme are regulated.

Yan-Qing Ye

(b 1906) Chinese orthopedic surgeon who did research on bone metabolism and microstructure, and surgery on fracture dislocation of the spine with cord injury.

Alexandre Émile John Yersin

(1863–1943) Swiss-born French microbiologist who, with Pasteur, discovered the causative agent of plague (*Yersinia pestis*) and developed a serum against it, worked on the diphtheria antitoxin, and founded two Pasteur institutes in China.

Hugh Young

(1870–1945) American urologist who invented procedures for intravesicular diverticulotomy, perineal prostatectomy, and for surgical treatment of retrourethral fistula.

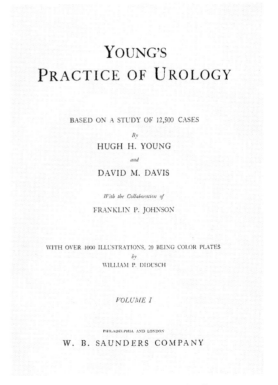

YOUNG'S
PRACTICE OF UROLOGY

BASED ON A STUDY OF 12,500 CASES
By
HUGH H. YOUNG
and
DAVID M. DAVIS

With the Collaboration of
FRANKLIN P. JOHNSON

WITH OVER 1000 ILLUSTRATIONS, 20 BEING COLOR PLATES
by
WILLIAM P. DIDUSCH

VOLUME I

PHILADELPHIA AND LONDON
W. B. SAUNDERS COMPANY

Title page from Young's book

Thomas Young

(1773–1829) Brilliant British physician and polymath, founder of physiological optics, who wrote *On the Mechanism of the Eye*, described astigmatism and accommodation, color vision and color blindness, and developed the wave theory of light.

Jean Yperman

(1295–1351) Belgian surgeon who performed ligation and torsion of arteries, described trephining, arrow wounds, harelip surgery, and used a silver tube for artificial feeding.

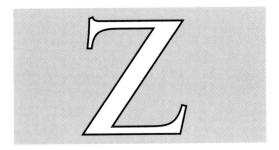

Gabriele Zerbi

(1468–1505) Italian anatomist who wrote an anatomic treatise that first separated organs into systems, described the muscles of the stomach, and the punta lachrymalia.

Norton David Zinder

(b 1928) American geneticist who discovered bacterial transduction – transfer of a gene from one bacterium to another by a phage – thus providing an explanation for the spread of drug resistance in bacteria and a method for inserting genes into bacteria.

Rolf M Zinkernagel

(b 1944) Swiss immunologist, pathologist and Nobel laureate who worked on the mechanism whereby the immune system T lymphocytes distinguishes virus-infected cells from normal cells.

Hans Zinsser

(1878–1940) American microbiologist who differentiated epidemic and endemic forms of the rickettsial disease typhus, wrote *Rats, Lice and History*, and studied allergy, rheumatic fever and the measurement of virus size.

Bernhard Zondek

(1891–1967) German-born Israeli gynecologist and endocrinologist who developed (with Selmar Aschheim) the first reliable pregnancy test in 1928, and discovered that hormones from the anterior pituitary gland stimulated other endocrine glands to release their hormones.

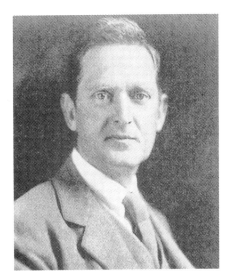

Hans Zinsser

Yvunge Zotterman

(1898–1982) Swedish physician who wrote a two-volume autobiography *Touch, Tickle and Pain*, describing his research on nerve impulses, sensory function of skin, and taste.